Contents

Preface *vii*
Symbols and abbreviations *ix*
Contributors *xi*

1. Epidemiology, pathology, and pathophysiology
   Graham S. Devereux   1

2. Diagnosis
   Graeme P. Currie   13

3. Non-pharmacological management
   Graeme P. Currie and John F.W. Baker   27

4. Pharmacological management
   Graeme P. Currie   37

5. Inhalers
   Graeme P. Currie   55

6. Acute exacerbations
   John F.W. Baker and Graeme P. Currie   65

7. Occupational asthma
   Edward W. Paterson and Graeme P. Currie   79

8. Asthma in special circumstances
   *Pratheega Mahendra, John F.W. Baker
   and Graeme P. Currie*   87

9. Paediatric asthma: epidemiology and aetiology
   Steve Turner   95

10. Paediatric asthma: diagnosis
    Steve Turner   101

11. Paediatric asthma: acute management
    Steve Turner   107

12. Paediatric asthma: chronic management
    Steve Turner   113

13. Asthma in primary care
    Cathy M. Jackson   123

14. Difficult asthma
    Claire A. Butler and Liam G. Heaney   131

    Index *141*

Preface

Asthma is a common chronic inflammatory condition affecting the airways and displays a varied phenotypic picture. It is becoming increasingly recognized by health care workers and epidemiological studies suggest that along with other atopic diseases its prevalence is rising. The precise aetiology of asthma remains uncertain, but genetic and environmental factors such as viruses, country of origin, allergen exposure, early use of antibiotics, and numbers of siblings have all been implicated in its inception and development. Pathologically it is characterized by inflammation, physiologically by airway hyper responsiveness (or hyper reactivity) resulting in reversible airflow obstruction, and clinically by wheeze, chest tightness, breathlessness and cough. It can present in early childhood as well as adulthood, and varies markedly in severity, clinical course, subsequent disability and response to treatment. Exacerbations and symptoms of asthma are the final manifestation of a complex interplay between an array of inflammatory cells and mediators, which cause airway smooth muscle to intermittently relax and contract.

Despite greater knowledge surrounding the immunopathological origins of asthma and considerable advances in its management, it remains one of the most important chronic diseases in young Western adults and poses a significant degree of morbidity throughout all age groups. A minority of patients have difficult to control asthma and often pose significant therapeutic difficulties in specialist clinics. Exacerbations of asthma contribute to significant costs for health care systems and are implicated in adversely affecting the quality of life of individuals and their families. Moreover, although asthma deaths have decreased over the past few decades, an appreciable number of deaths still occur each year. Regular anti-inflammatory therapy with ICSs is required in all but the mildest of disease and attenuates underlying airway inflammation and hyper responsiveness, while bronchodilators are designed to relax airway smooth muscle and prevent bronchoconstriction on exposure to bronchoconstrictor stimuli. Other forms of treatment are required in individuals with persistent symptoms and exacerbations. The aim of this book is to offer a compact, practical, contemporary and referenced evidence based guide by which to offer the reader a useful update of the main clinical aspects of the overall syndrome of asthma.

Symbols and abbreviations

ACE	angiotensin converting enzyme
BTS/SIGN	British Thoracic Society/Scottish Intercollegiate Guidelines Network (BTS/SIGN)
COPD	chronic obstructive pulmonary disease
COSHH	Control of Substances Hazardous to Health
DPI	Dry powder inhalers
FEV_1	forced expiratory volume in 1 second
FVC	forced vital capacity
HADS	Hospital Anxiety and Depression Scale
ICS	inhaled corticosteroids
LABA	long acting β_2-agonist
LTRA	leukotriene receptor antagonist
MDI	metered dose inhaler
NIV	non-invasive ventilation
NSAID	non-steroidal anti-inflammatory drugs
OASYS	Occupational Asthma Expert System
pANCA	serum p anti-neutrophil cytoplasmic antibody
PEF	peak expiratory flow
pMDI	pressurised metered dose inhalers
QOF	Quality Outcome Framework
RADS	reactive airways dysfunction syndrome
RIDDOR	Reporting of Injuries, Diseases and Dangerous Occurrences Regulations
RISA	Research in Severe Asthma
SABA	short acting beta agonist
SMART	Single Maintenance And Reliever Therapy

Contributors

John F.W. Baker, MBChB, BA (Hons)
Foundation Doctor, Aberdeen Royal Infirmary, Aberdeen, Scotland, UK

Claire A. Butler, MB BCh, BAO, MRCP (UK), PhD
Belfast City Hospital, Belfast, Northern Ireland, UK

Graeme P. Currie, MBChB, DCH, Pg Dip M Ed, MD, FRCP (Ed)
Consultant Respiratory Physician, Aberdeen Royal Infirmary, Aberdeen, Scotland, UK

Graham S. Devereux, MBChB, MA, MD, PhD, FRCP(Ed)
Clinical Senior Lecturer, Honorary Consultant Physician, Department of Environmental and Occupational Medicine, University of Aberdeen, Aberdeen, Scotland, UK

Liam G. Heaney, MBChB, MRCP, MD
Consultant Respiratory Physician, Belfast City Hospital, Belfast, Northern Ireland, UK

Cathy M. Jackson, BSc (Hons), MBChB, MRCGP, MD
Clinical Senior Lecturer, Community Health Sciences, University of Dundee, Dundee, Scotland, UK

Edward W. Paterson, MBChB, MRCP (UK), Pg Dip M Ed
Locum Consultant Respiratory Physician, Aberdeen Royal Infirmary, Aberdeen, Scotland, UK

Pratheega Mahendra, MBChB, MRCP (UK)
Specialist Registrar in Respiratory Medicine, Aberdeen Royal Infirmary, Aberdeen, Scotland, UK

Steve Turner, MBBS, MRCP, FRCPCH, MD
Consultant Paediatrician, Royal Hospital for Sick Children, Aberdeen, Scotland, UK

Chapter 1

Epidemiology, pathology, and pathophysiology

Graham S. Devereux

> **Key points**
>
> - Asthma is more common in affluent Westernized countries and its prevalence has increased over the last 40 years
> - Features associated with a Westernized lifestyle such as improved hygiene, obesity and diet have been suggested as possible contributory causes to the rise in allergic diseases such as asthma
> - Asthma is more prevalent in children (10–15%) than adults (5–10%); in children, it is more common in males and in adults more common in females
> - A genetic tendency along with environmental influences leads to hallmark features of asthma, which are inflammation, airway hyperresponsiveness and reversible airflow obstruction.

1.1 Definition

Although asthma has been described in literature since antiquity, the condition effectively remains undefined. No single parameter can be used to diagnose asthma with certainty; consequently asthma remains a clinical diagnosis. A 1992 International Consensus Report described asthma as:

> a chronic inflammatory disorder of the airways in which many cells play a role, in particular mast cells and eosinophils. In susceptible individuals, this inflammation causes symptoms which are usually associated with widespread but variable airflow obstruction that is often reversible either spontaneously or with treatment and causes an associated increase in airway responsiveness to a variety of stimuli.

The absence of specific defining criteria limits the interpretation of epidemiological and pathophysiological studies, that have used different methods to identify subjects with asthma. Studies that have used a clinical diagnosis of asthma to identify subjects are liable to subtle yet important inconsistencies due to variation in access, provision and quality of healthcare services and international differences in the diagnostic practices of doctors. Public awareness of asthma also appears to heavily influence the prevalence of asthma reported in a population.

1.2 **Epidemiology**

Asthma is one of the world's most common chronic diseases with a conservative estimate of 300 million people suffering from it globally. It is estimated that by 2025 there could be an additional 100 million people with the disease worldwide.

1.2.1 **Geographical differences**

International surveys that have used standardized methodologies demonstrate marked geographical variation in the prevalence of asthma and asthma symptoms both within and between countries. Studies of children and adults report high prevalence rates (15–20%) in the United Kingdom, Australia, New Zealand and other developed countries and low (2–4%) rates in Asian countries (especially China and India).

Studies of migratory populations, and those performed after the reunification of Germany, clearly demonstrate that exposure to an affluent Westernized lifestyle, particularly during early childhood is associated with an increased likelihood of developing asthma and allergic disease. In less well developed areas such as Africa, the prevalence among rural African children living a traditional lifestyle in the 1970s was very low when compared to urban children. However, recent studies indicate that this rural/urban gap—while still present—has narrowed appreciably. This has been attributed to an increasing tendency for rural communities to adopt a more Westernized lifestyle.

1.2.2 **Age and sex differences**

Asthma is more common in children than adults, although of these, between 30% and 80% of children become asymptomatic around the time of puberty. Longitudinal cohort studies suggest complex and somewhat unpredictable associations between childhood asthma and asthma status during adult life. About a quarter of children continue to have the condition as adults and about a quarter of children who undergo remission during puberty relapse as adults. Furthermore, about 10% of children who have never wheezed will develop wheezing as adults. In childhood, asthma is more prevalent in males, but during puberty the sex ratio reverses such that asthma is more common in females. There is some evidence to suggest a further reversal of the sex ratio after the age of 50 years when asthma is probably more common in males.

1.2.3 Temporal trends

There is convincing evidence that the prevalence of asthma markedly increased in Westernized countries between the 1960s and the 1990s. While this may in part reflect the increasing awareness of family doctors of asthma, repeated cross-sectional surveys consistently report increases in wheezing illness and objective parameters of asthma such as airway hyperresponsiveness. Some of the recent increases may be secondary to the rise in atopic diseases (atopic eczema, allergic rhinitis) that are recognized risk factors for the development of asthma (Figures 1.1 and 1.2). Since the 1990s there is evidence that whilst the prevalence of asthma has continued to increase in some countries, in others it has been stable and in some it has declined.

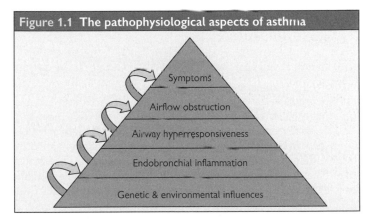

Figure 1.1 The pathophysiological aspects of asthma

Symptoms

Airflow obstruction

Airway hyperresponsiveness

Endobronchial inflammation

Genetic & environmental influences

1.2.4 Impact of asthma

In Westernized countries, asthma is now a major public health concern; it is common and associated with significant ill health and high societal and healthcare costs.

In the UK, 10–15% of children and 5–10% of adults have been diagnosed with asthma and it has been estimated that 5.2 million individuals receive treatment for asthma, of whom 1.1 million are children. However, despite the large numbers of affected individuals, the mortality rate is low; around 1,400 deaths were attributed to asthma in the UK in 2002, with more than two-thirds being aged 65 years or older.

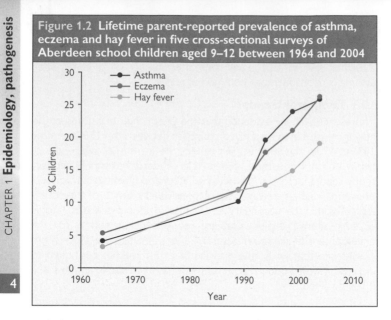

Figure 1.2 Lifetime parent-reported prevalence of asthma, eczema and hay fever in five cross-sectional surveys of Aberdeen school children aged 9–12 between 1964 and 2004

Asthma is associated with significant morbidity with an estimated 2.1 million adults and 500,000 children experiencing frequent severe symptoms, while one in six individuals experience weekly exacerbations such that they have difficulty speaking. Moreover, 6% of asthmatics require emergency treatment every month. Individuals with asthma are significant consumers of NHS resources and services, particularly in primary care. In the UK in 2000, there were more than 18,000 first new episodes presenting to general practitioners, and there are over 4 million consultations with general practitioners annually. In 2002 there were 69,000 admissions to hospital in the UK because of asthma; admission rates for adults have remained stable over the past few years. The annual UK economic cost of asthma in 2001 was estimated to be £2.3 billion, with the 12.7 million working days that were lost annually accounting for £1.2 billion in lost productivity. A further £260 million was accounted for by social security benefits and NHS expenditure on asthma was estimated to be £889 million (Figure 1.3). In the United States, between 2001 and 2003 there were an average of 20 million people with asthma, with 6.2 million of them being children. The most recent estimates of the economic burden of asthma in the United States in 2007 reported that the total economic cost of asthma to society was $56 billion annually, with $3.8 billion being accounted for by lost productivity due to ill-health and $2.1 billion lost in productivity because of mortality.

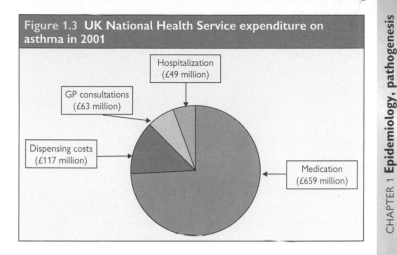

Figure 1.3 UK National Health Service expenditure on asthma in 2001

Hospitalization (£49 million)

GP consultations (£63 million)

Dispensing costs (£117 million)

Medication (£659 million)

1.3 Pathology

There is little doubt that asthma is an inflammatory condition of the airways. Post-mortem studies demonstrate that the lungs of individuals who have died from asthma are hyperinflated with widespread plugging of small, medium and, to some extent, large airways by thick tenacious mucus; there are also small areas of pulmonary atelectasis/collapse. The development of fibreoptic bronchoscopy with histological analysis of bronchial biopsies and cytological examination of bronchoalveolar lavage samples, has demonstrated that even mild asthma is associated with airway inflammation, albeit less severe than that observed in fatal disease.

Microscopically, asthma is associated with epithelial disruption with the shedding of epithelial cells into the airway lumen; clusters of epithelial cells form Creola bodies that can be identified in the sputum. Further characteristic features of asthmatic airways are homogeneous thickening of the subepithelial reticular basement membrane and an increase in smooth muscle mass as a consequence of hypertrophy and/or proliferation (Figure 1.4). Asthmatic airways tend to be inflamed and oedematous, and have dilated blood vessels, endothelial swelling and angiogenesis. Characteristically there is a marked cellular infiltrate of CD4+ T-helper (Th) lymphocytes of the Th2 phenotype, eosinophils and mast cells. Asthma is also associated with increased mucus production due to goblet cell hyperplasia and submucosal mucus gland hypertrophy. The excess of mucus, when mixed with inflammatory exudate, inflammatory cells and epithelial cells, form highly tenacious mucus plugs that are difficult to clear and contribute to airflow obstruction. The airway lumen is further

Figure 1.4 Schematic representation of the histopathological features of asthma

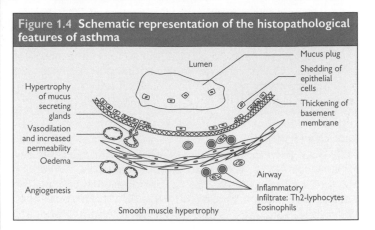

compromised by airway thickening associated with airway inflammation and dynamic airflow obstruction resulting from contraction of increased airway smooth muscle mass.

1.4 Pathophysiology

1.4.1 Lymphocytes

A major advance in the understanding of the immunopathology of asthma was the demonstration that CD4+ Th cells could be categorized into two broad functional groups (Th1 and Th2) based on their secreted cytokines. Asthma and allergic disease are associated with the Th2 phenotype characterized by the secretion of interleukin (IL) 4, IL-5, IL-6, IL-9, IL-10 and IL-13 (Figure 1.5). The Th2 cytokine IL-4 induces the isotype switching of B cells to the synthesis of IgE, and IL-5 promotes the growth, differentiation and release of eosinophils from bone marrow. IL-13 can also switch B cells to IgE secretion and increases airway mucus production through goblet cell hyperplasia. Other actions of Th2 cytokines include the growth, differentiation and release of mast cells from bone marrow, localization and activation of eosinophils, and inhibition of Th1 differentiation. Th2 biased Th cells induce a package of biological responses that are characteristic of asthma, allergy and helminth infection, namely high levels of circulating immunoglobulin E (IgE), mastocytosis and tissue eosinophilia.

In recent years regulatory T-cells that can suppress Th1 and Th2 differentiation and activity have been identified and implicated in asthma immunopathogenesis, with several studies reporting asthma to be associated with reduced numbers and activity of CD4$^+$, CD25$^+$, FoxP3$^+$ and IL-10 secreting regulatory T-cells. Further T-cells (natural killer, $\gamma\delta$, CD8) and Th-cell subsets (Th9, Th17, Th22) have been recently described and identified in asthma and/or mouse models of asthma. However, their role in asthma remains to be elucidated. Of particular interest is the concept that different T-cell and Th-cell subsets may be important in the various clinical manifestations of asthma, e.g. atopic asthma, non-atopic asthma, and steroid resistant asthma.

1.4.2 Eosinophils

Eosinophils are probably the major effector cells in asthma, with elevated numbers found in the sputum, airways and blood. Circulating eosinophils localize to inflamed airways by various adhesion molecules (such as intercellular adhesion molecule 1 (ICAM-1)) and chemokines (such as eotaxin) released by Th2 cells and inflammatory cells. Once localized to the airways, activated eosinophils release highly toxic granule proteins (e.g. eosinophil cationic protein and major basic protein) and free radicals that can kill parasites, but in the

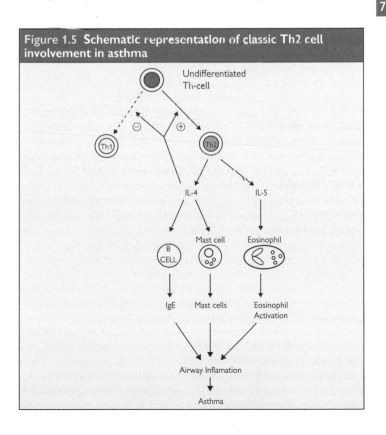

Figure 1.5 Schematic representation of classic Th2 cell involvement in asthma

inappropriate setting of asthma, cause tissue damage. The synthesis and release of inflammatory molecules such as prostaglandins, leukotrienes and cytokines amplify and perpetuate the inflammatory response by further recruitment of eosinophils and lymphocytes.

1.4.3 Immunoglobulin E

Elevated IgE levels are a feature of atopic/allergic asthma and IgE mediates allergen-induced bronchoconstriction. The IgE stimulated by Th2 biased responses is specific for the stimulating antigen (pollens, animal or insect dander) and most is bound to tissue mast cells, which possess high affinity FcɛR1 receptors on their cell surface. Exposure of IgE-coated mast cells to specific multivalent antigen induces mast cell activation by cross-linkage of the IgE molecules. Mast cell activation induces the rapid (within seconds) release of preformed (histamine, tryptase, chymase) and rapidly synthesized mediators (prostaglandins, leukotrienes). These inflammatory mediators induce bronchoconstriction, mucus secretion, vasodilatation, nerve stimulation, increased vascular permeability, tissue oedema and eosinophil chemotaxis. Activated mast cells also secrete cytokines and chemokines that promote Th2 differentiation and the influx of lymphocytes and eosinophils. Allergen-induced, IgE-mediated mast cell activation induces a characteristic rapid inflammatory response known as the immediate hypersensitivity reaction. The immediate response is rapid and intense, but short lived because of rapid degradation of inflammatory mediators. In some individuals, the immediate response is followed 4–8 hours later by a slowly developing, intense and sustained response, known as the late phase reaction. The sustained late phase response is often considered to be the pathophysiological basis for the chronic allergic inflammatory state found in asthma. The late phase response is initiated by mast cell degranulation of the immediate hypersensitivity reaction, which releases inflammatory mediators that recruit and activate eosinophils, neutrophils, basophils, macrophages and Th2 cells, which release further inflammatory mediators that induce the late phase response (Figure 1.6). Once the inflammatory state has been established in asthma, the airways demonstrate an increased propensity to constrict in response to non-allergenic stimuli such as exercise, cold air and pollution. This is known as bronchial hyperresponsiveness or hyperreactivity and is believed to be the mechanism behind spontaneous and induced variability of airflow obstruction.

1.4.4 Remodelling of airways

Asthma is associated with structural changes of the airways (thickened basement membrane, smooth muscle hypertrophy), and in an important subgroup of individuals with asthma there is an accelerated decline in ventilatory function. This phenomenon of airway

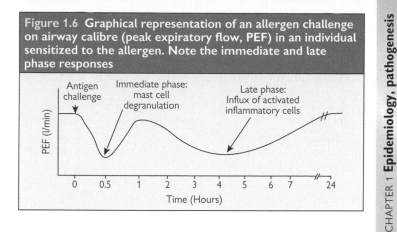

Figure 1.6 Graphical representation of an allergen challenge on airway calibre (peak expiratory flow, PEF) in an individual sensitized to the allergen. Note the immediate and late phase responses

remodelling has conventionally been thought to be a consequence of chronic airway inflammation. However, there is emerging evidence suggesting that airway remodelling is an independent parallel process fundamental to asthma that commences very early in life, perhaps even *in utero*. The shedding of epithelial cells is a characteristic feature of asthma and normally the integrity of the surface epithelium is rapidly restored. However, there is evidence to suggest that in asthma the epithelium is not only more susceptible to environmental stressors (air pollution, viruses, oxidative stress) but that the proliferative repair response to restore epithelial integrity is defective. It has been suggested that increased airway epithelial susceptibility and defective repair stimulates the persistent activation and secretion of inflammatory epithelial-derived cytokines and growth factors that interact with immune cells and drives chronic inflammation and remodelling of the subepithelial compartment.

1.5 **Risk factors for asthma**

Asthma develops in individuals because of a combination of genetic predisposition and environmental exposures. It also seems highly likely that the contributory effects of these predisposing factors to the development of asthma differ at differing times of life.

1.5.1 **Genetic factors**
A well-established clinical observation is that asthma and allergic disease run in families and that, in an individual, the presence of one of these conditions increases the likelihood of related conditions. Formal investigations have confirmed this clinical observation and twin studies suggest that 50–60% of asthma is inherited.

In recent years many associations have been reported between polymorphisms in genes encoding for molecules implicated in the immunopathogenesis of asthma and allergy. Many of these associations have now been replicated. A number of chromosome regions containing clusters of biologically relevant genes for asthma have been reported. Examples include a cytokine cluster on chromosome 5q, the gene for the β chain of the high affinity receptor for IgE (FCER1B) on 11q, the genes for interferon-γ and the signalling molecule STAT6 on 12q and the α-chain of the IL-4 receptor on 16p. Other genes that have been linked with asthma and replicated include ADAM33 a protein implicated in airway development and remodelling, GPRA, a molecule expressed in airway smooth muscle and epithelial cells and the $β_2$-adrenoceptor gene (ADRB2).

1.5.2 **Exposure to tobacco smoke**

Maternal cigarette smoking during pregnancy has been consistently associated with an increased risk of childhood wheezing disease and asthma. Antenatal exposure to tobacco smoke has been reported to be associated with reduced neonatal lung function and altered neonatal immunity. Of particular interest has been the recent demonstration of a so called 'grandmother' effect whereby maternal smoking during pregnancy not only increases the risk of asthma in her children, but also in the children born to her daughters. Such a transgenerational effect of smoking may be a consequence of epigenetic modification of germ cell genes in the developing female fetus.

1.5.3 **Allergen exposure**

Allergen exposure and IgE sensitization to allergens are central to the understanding of the immunopathogenesis of asthma, and sensitization to perennial allergens such as house dust mite is associated with an increased likelihood of asthma. However, a meta-analysis of trials of early life allergen (dust mite, specific foods) avoidance demonstrate that allergen avoidance does not reduce the likelihood of childhood asthma.

1.5.4 **Hygiene**

The hygiene hypothesis proposes that the development of asthma and allergic disease is increased by a lack of exposure to infections and microbial products because of improved hygiene, cleanliness and widespread antibiotic use, common in Westernized societies. Studies of children born and brought up on farms demonstrate that they are less likely to develop asthma and allergic disease. This so called 'farming effect' appears to be a consequence of maternal exposure to the farming environment during pregnancy, with a higher burden and diversity of microbial contamination of the environment appearing to be beneficial. Such exposures of pregnant women to microbial structural molecules such as endotoxins appear to affect the developing immune system of the fetus.

1.5.5 Obesity and inactivity

The recent increase in asthma and allergic disease in Westernized countries has been paralleled by an increase in obesity and it has been hypothesized that obesity is a risk factor for asthma in children and adults. Longitudinal studies have demonstrated that being overweight increases the likelihood of developing asthma by about 40% and being obese by about 90%. The mechanism underlying this association is an area of active research. Although obesity adversely affects lung mechanics, cardiovascular function and increases gastro-oesophageal reflux there is increasing interest in the concept that the airway inflammation of asthma is a manifestation of the systematic inflammatory state associated with obesity.

1.5.6 Diet

Many studies have demonstrated associations between asthma and dietary intake of antioxidants (vitamin C, vitamin E, B-carotene, selenium), polyunsaturated fatty acids (n-3, n-6) and some foodstuffs (apples, fruit juice, butter, margarine). However, dietary supplementation in adults is not associated with any clinically beneficial effect. A number of recent studies have highlighted the potentially important role of maternal diet during pregnancy in influencing the likelihood of childhood asthma, in particular, the consumption of vitamin E, vitamin D, zinc, n-3 polyunsaturated fatty acids and apples. Further studies are required before firm recommendations can be made.

1.5.7 Occupation

It has been estimated that in the UK about 9–15% of adult onset asthma is a consequence of occupational exposure. There are over 400 reported causes of occupational asthma and about 90% of occupational asthma is a consequence of allergic sensitization to the occupational sensitizing agent. The most frequent causative occupational exposures include isocyanates (paint spraying), flour/grain dust (bakers, pastry makers), colophony/fluxes (welders), latex (healthcare workers), animals (animal handlers) and wood dust (timber workers).

1.5.8 Outdoor air pollution

Ambient levels of air pollutants such as particulates, oxides of nitrogen and sulphur dioxide have an adverse effect on established asthma, and are associated with increased rates of exacerbations and hospitalization. Whether air pollution increases the risk of developing asthma is less clear. The increase in asthma and allergic diseases in the latter decades of the 20th century occurred at the same time as air pollution declined in the UK. There is evidence of an adverse association between the incidence of asthma and levels of particulates and oxides of nitrogen in children living very close to busy roads, especially if traffic includes heavy goods vehicles. However, the proportion of children living close to such roads is small and consequently at a population level, there is no association between the incidence of asthma and air pollution.

Further reading

Allan K, Devereux G. (2011) Diet and asthma: nutritional implications from prevention to treatment. *J Am Dietetic Ass*, **111**: 258–68.

Asthma UK (2004) *Where Do We Stand?* http://www.asthma.org.uk/ document. rm?id=18 (accessed 8/11).

Crane J, von Mutius E, Custovic A (2006) Epidemiology of allergic disease. In: *Allergy*, 3rd edn (eds Holgate ST, Church MK, Litchenstein LM), pp. 233–246. Elsevier St. Louis.

International consensus report on diagnosis and treatment of asthma (1992) National Heart, Lung, and Blood Institute, National Institutes of Health, Bethesda, Maryland 20892. Publication No. 92–3091, March 1992. *Eur Respir J*, **5**: 601–41.

Jeffrey PK (2001) Remodelling in asthma and chronic obstructive lung disease. *Am J Respir Crit Care Med*, **164**: S28–S38.

Meyers DA (2010) Genetics of asthma and allergy: what have we learned? *J Allergy Clin Immunol*, **126**: 439–46.

Van Schayck OCP, Maas T, Kaper J, Knottnerus AJA, Sheikh A (2007) Is there any role for allergen avoidance in the primary prevention of childhood asthma? *J Allergy Clin Immunol*, **119**: 1328–8.

Chapter 2

Diagnosis

Graeme P. Currie

Key points

- The diagnosis of asthma is based around the presence of typical symptoms (intermittent cough, wheeze, breathlessness, impaired exercise tolerance, chest tightness) and assessment of spirometry
- In asthma, spirometry is usually normal, although airflow obstruction may be present
- Depending on clinical features and spirometry, the probability of asthma being present should be categorized into high, intermediate or low:
  - High probability: treatment should be started
  - Intermediate probability: treatment should be started if spirometry is normal or airflow obstruction present; otherwise, further investigations and an alternative diagnosis should be considered
  - Low probability: further investigations and an alternative diagnosis should be considered
- Further investigations may include a full blood count, reversibility testing, exercise testing, chest X-ray, and assessment of airway hyperresponsiveness, exhaled nitric oxide, and sputum eosinophils.

13

2.1 Diagnosis

Making the diagnosis of asthma is not always straightforward. Unlike many other conditions in medicine, the diagnosis is usually based on typical features in the history along with assessment of spirometry, with no discriminatory examination, radiological or laboratory findings. It is important to identify key features in the history, carry out a careful physical examination and perform spirometry and thereby determine whether patients have a high, intermediate or low probability of asthma. Based on this probability, management options will include a trial of treatment, or the consideration of an alternative diagnosis and further investigations. (Figure 2.1).

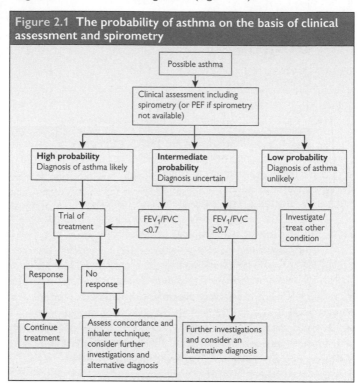

Figure 2.1 The probability of asthma on the basis of clinical assessment and spirometry

2.1.1 Clinical features and differential diagnosis

Classical features of asthma include wheeze, chest tightness, breathlessness, reduced exercise tolerance and cough. These may occur in isolation or combination. Asthma is more likely if symptoms appear following exercise, exposure to cold air, aspirin, β-blockers and allergens, or occur overnight or early in the morning. Examples of other provoking stimuli include:

- Respiratory infections
- Cigarette smoke
- Stress and anxiety
- Pets and furry animals
- Grass, weed, and tree pollens
- Drugs, e.g. β-blockers (including eye drops), non-steroidal anti-inflammatory drugs (NSAIDs), and aspirin
- Food additives, e.g. tartrazine, benzoates
- Environmental and occupational agents.

Clinical features which make asthma *more* likely include:

- Past or current history of atopic disorders
- Family history of asthma or atopic disorders
- Otherwise unexplained peripheral blood eosinophilia
- Otherwise unexplained reduced FEV_1 or PEF.

Factors that make asthma *less* likely include:

- Voice disturbance
- Dizziness, lightheadedness or tingling
- Productive cough with wheeze or breathlessness
- Normal chest examination when symptomatic
- Normal FEV_1 or PEF when symptomatic.

Particular respiratory symptoms are neither sensitive nor specific for the diagnosis of asthma. Examples of disorders that can mimic symptoms of asthma and enter the differential diagnosis include:

- Chronic obstructive pulmonary disease (COPD)
- Hyperventilation
- Angiotensin converting enzyme (ACE) inhibitor induced cough
- Vocal cord dysfunction
- Bronchiectasis
- Cystic fibrosis
- Chronic idiopathic syndromes
- Interstitial lung disease
- Chronic pulmonary thromboembolic disease
- Lung cancer
- Pulmonary hypertension
- Upper airway obstruction (e.g. vocal cord palsy, cancer, tracheomalacia, tracheal stenosis)
- Pulmonary oedema
- Sarcoidosis
- Breathlessness due to obesity or anaemia.

Of all these conditions, COPD is often in the main differential diagnosis for asthma in adults with a smoking history. Distinguishing between these two conditions is not always straightforward (Table 2.1). Clinicians should, however, endeavour to do so, as both have different treatments and prognosis. In some individuals, there is a degree of overlap between asthma and COPD.

Twin and familial studies suggest a genetic link in asthma and it is important to discover if other family members are known to be affected. Other atopic diseases commonly coexist with asthma and clinicians should therefore enquire about a personal history of allergic rhinitis and eczema. Indeed, allergic rhinitis is found to some

Table 2.1 Clinical features that help distinguish asthma from chronic obstructive pulmonary disease (COPD)

	Asthma	COPD
Age	Any age	>35 years
Cough	Often non-productive	Frequently productive
Breathlessness	Episodic	Persistent and progressive
Atopic disorders	Common	Possible
Family history	Frequent	No link
Smoking history	Possible	Almost invariable
Lung function	Often normal	Always abnormal

extent in many patients with allergic asthma; many studies have demonstrated that patients who have been treated for allergic rhinitis experience fewer exacerbations of asthma. This in turn highlights the importance of asking about symptoms such as nasal obstruction and discharge, post-nasal drip, impaired smell, chronic cough and repeated throat clearing.

2.1.2 Signs

All patients in whom the diagnosis of asthma is suspected should be examined. The examination is often completely normal but it is important to identify features that may indicate a concomitant or alternative diagnosis. Evidence of allergic rhinitis or eczema may also be found in a proportion of individuals. Patients may only have demonstrable signs—such as wheeze—during an exacerbation or following exposure to a particular trigger due to the variable nature of the condition.

2.1.3 Spirometry

Spirometry is indicated in all individuals with suspected asthma. This involves the patient performing a forced respiratory manoeuvre, which measures forced expiratory volume in 1 second (FEV_1), forced vital capacity (FVC) and the FEV_1/FVC ratio. Due to the variable nature of asthma, spirometry may be normal. However, airflow obstruction may be present during an exacerbation or when symptoms are undertreated. In more severe asthma, the FVC may become impaired, which may indicate the development of more fixed airways disease. Table 2.2 shows the typical features of normal, obstructive, restrictive and mixed obstructive/restrictive spirometry. Table 2.3 shows different causes of obstructive and restrictive ventilatory defects.

Table 2.2 Features of normal, obstructive, restrictive, and mixed obstructive/restrictive spirometry

Pattern	FEV_1	FVC	FEV_1/FVC
Normal	≥80% predicted	≥80% predicted	0.7–0.8
Obstructive	<80% predicted	>80% predicted (or <80% predicted in advanced disease)	<0.7
Restrictive	<80% predicted	<80% predicted (FEV_1 and FVC are reduced proportionally)	≥0.7
Mixed obstructive/ restrictive	<80% predicted	<80% predicted (FEV_1 is reduced to a greater extent than FVC)	<0.7

Table 2.3 Causes of obstructive and restrictive spirometry

Obstructive	Restrictive
Asthma	Pulmonary fibrosis
COPD	Kyphoscoliosis
Bronchiectasis	Morbid obesity
	Large pleural effusion
	Previous pneumonectomy
	Neuromuscular disorders

Based on clinical features and spirometry, the probability of asthma should be stratified into high, intermediate or low probabilities (Figure 2.1). Depending on this, treatment should be initiated or an alternative diagnosis and additional tests considered.

2.2 **Other investigations**

If response to treatment is poor, or if the probability of asthma is intermediate or low, a variety of different investigations can be considered.

2.2.1 **Reversibility testing**

If airflow obstruction is present and the probability of a diagnosis of asthma is intermediate or low, it may be appropriate to look for objective evidence of reversibility. Reversibility testing can be performed using either B_2-agonists or corticosteroids. The FEV_1 or PEF is recorded initially and then 20 minutes following a short-acting

B$_2$-agonist (SABA) delivered via a nebulizer (2.5 mg salbutamol) or hand-held inhaler (200 micrograms or 2 puffs of salbutamol). Alternatively, patients may be given a trial of oral corticosteroid (such as prednisolone 30 mg daily for 2 weeks) or 400 micrograms of inhaled Beclometasone for 6 weeks. In all of these methods, an improvement in FEV$_1$ >20% or 400ml from baseline, or increase in PEF by 60 l/min is highly suggestive of asthma.

2.2.2 **Variability in peak expiratory flow**

Assessing the variability in peak expiratory flow (PEF) over several weeks is now less commonly used to diagnose asthma, as its sensitivity is low. However, it is still used in the diagnosis of occupational asthma and assessing the degree of asthma control. PEF is a measure of the maximal rate of exhalation. In normal adults, it peaks at the age of 30 and varies according to height, sex, race and age. If the PEF is normal when a patient has symptoms, then it is less likely that asthma is present. To correctly use a peak flow meter (Figure 2.2), the following steps should be followed:

- Set the pointer to zero
- Inhale to total lung capacity
- Seal the lips around the mouthpiece
- Exhale as hard and fast as possible
- Record the number next to the pointer.

Box 2.1 How to calculate the percentage variability

Variability = (best PEF−lowest PEF)/best PEF x 100

For example,

- Highest PEF = 500 L/min
- Lowest PEF = 400 L/min
- Variation in PEF = 500 L/min−400 L/min = 100 L/min
- % PEF variability = (500−400)/500 x 100 = 20%

Figure 2.2 PEF meter

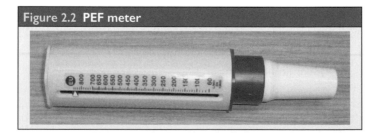

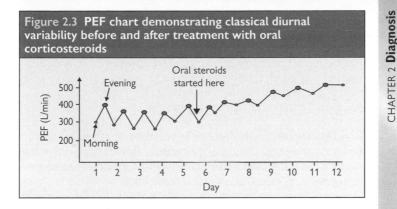

Figure 2.3 PEF chart demonstrating classical diurnal variability before and after treatment with oral corticosteroids

The PEF should be taken first thing in the morning, last thing in the evening, and sometimes in between these times; the best of three attempts should be recorded into a peak flow diary. A 20% difference in PEF recordings during three consecutive days during a week over a 2-week period may be consistent with the diagnosis of asthma (Figure 2.3; Box 2.1).

2.2.3 **Exercise testing**

Many patients—typically those with normal lung function—do not demonstrate significant reversibility following an inhaled acting β_2-agonist or course of oral prednisolone. In these patients an exercise test may be performed. PEF is measured at rest and the patient performs high intensity exercise (e.g. running) for 6 minutes. The PEF is then recorded every 10 minutes for 30 minutes; a fall of 20% is considered consistent with the diagnosis (Figure 2.4).

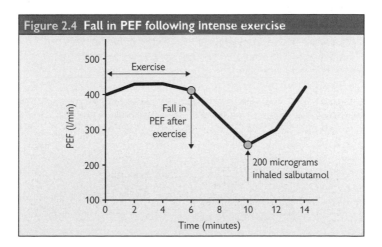

Figure 2.4 Fall in PEF following intense exercise

2.2.4 **Bronchial challenge testing**

Bronchial challenge tests can be used to assess the extent of airway hyperresponsiveness in asthma but are not routinely used in its diagnosis. The most commonly agents used are methacholine and histamine, both of which act directly upon receptors in bronchial smooth muscle and cause contraction leading to bronchoconstriction. However, inhalation of such stimuli can also cause bronchoconstriction in non-asthmatic individuals, those with COPD and smokers. Bronchoprovocation with indirect stimuli such as adenosine monophosphate, mannitol and hypertonic saline—which cause the initial release of proinflammatory mediators—are more closely associated with underlying inflammation than direct stimuli.

Most methods of assessing the degree of airway hyperresponsiveness follow the same general principles. An initial FEV_1 baseline is measured prior to administration of a bronchoconstrictor stimulus. Bronchoprovocation is then carried out using doubling doses or concentrations of the stimulus. At regular intervals (usually several minutes), the best of several FEV_1 measurements is recorded. The test is usually terminated after a predetermined fall in FEV_1 is achieved (usually a 20% fall). Construction of a log dose—response curve is followed by linear interpolation. This allows the provocative dose or concentration of stimulant to be calculated. The provocative dose or concentration of agent causing a 20% fall in FEV_1 is usually abbreviated to PD_{20} or PC_{20} (Figure 2.5). Patients can be given a SABA to quicken their return to pre-test value or allowed to recover spontaneously. Guidelines have suggested stratifying the degree of airway hyperresponsiveness to methacholine according to the PC_{20} value (Table 2.4).

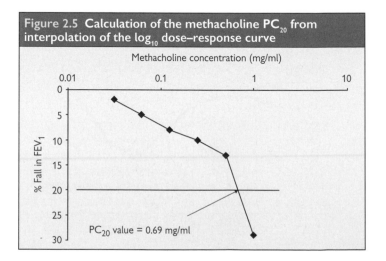

Figure 2.5 Calculation of the methacholine PC_{20} from interpolation of the log_{10} dose–response curve

Table 2.4 Severity of airway hyperresponsiveness according to the methacholine PC_{20}	
Extent of airway hyperresponsiveness	**Methacholine PC_{20}**
Absent	>16 mg/ml
Borderline	4–16 mg/ml
Mild	1–4 mg/ml
Moderate to severe	<1 mg/ml

Bronchial challenge tests tend to be reserved for research purposes in specialized centres, but may also be of value when diagnosis is uncertain. Patients who fail to demonstrate airway hyperresponsiveness despite significant symptoms should have the diagnosis of asthma reconsidered.

2.2.5 **Inflammatory biomarkers**

Inflammatory biomarkers such as sputum eosinophilia (Figure 2.6) and exhaled nitric oxide are of increasing interest in determining the presence and extent of airway inflammation. A differential sputum eosinophilia of >2% is found in many asthmatics and falls after anti-inflammatory treatment. It can be measured by asking patients to expectorate following treatment with inhaled hypertonic saline, although doing so can be time consuming and cumbersome.

Nitric oxide is produced predominantly within bronchial epithelial cells and an inducible isoform of nitric oxide synthase can be expressed in response to inflammation. This leads to the manufacture of increased levels of exhaled nitric oxide which can be measured within minutes

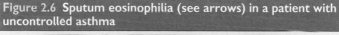
Figure 2.6 Sputum eosinophilia (see arrows) in a patient with uncontrolled asthma

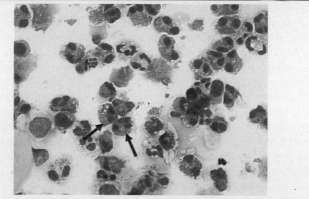

using hand-held analyzers. In untreated asthma, the exhaled nitric oxide level is typically >25 parts per billion, although levels can also be elevated in conditions other than asthma.

Titrating asthma therapy according to lung function and surrogate inflammatory biomarkers may lead to a more superior control of asthma symptoms than using lung function alone. Inflammatory biomarkers such as sputum eosinophils and exhaled nitric oxide are used increasingly in specialist clinics in an attempt to help confirm or refute the diagnosis of asthma. They are also commonly used in clinical trials evaluating the effects of anti-inflammatory treatment in asthma.

2.2.6 **Other investigations**

A chest radiograph may be required if an alternative diagnosis is considered or if patients have atypical symptoms or signs. A full blood count may also be useful, looking for the presence of a raised eosinophil count which is in keeping with the diagnosis of asthma. Skin prick tests or a radioallergosorbent test (RAST) may also be performed to identify whether individuals are sensitive to specific allergens, while an increased immunoglobulin E (IgE) level indicates that the individual is atopic.

2.3 **Asthma subtypes and associated syndromes**

2.3.1 **Allergic rhinitis**

Allergic rhinitis is a common inflammatory condition of the upper airway characterized by sneezing, nasal pruritus, rhinorrhoea, and nasal obstruction. Since the upper and lower airways have a direct anatomical connection, share similar epithelial lining, and release similar inflammatory mediators, it has been suggested that asthma and allergic rhinitis represent a continuation of the same inflammatory disease process.

Around 20–40% of individuals with allergic rhinitis are thought to have concomitant asthma, while 30–90% of asthmatics are thought to have allergic rhinitis. Uncontrolled allergic rhinitis is known to precipitate and exacerbate asthma, with the inference that clinicians should positively search for typical nasal and ocular symptoms. Moreover, successful treatment of allergic rhinitis can confer benefits in overall asthma control. Recent guidelines have emphasized the importance of identifying symptoms of asthma in individuals with rhinitis and vice versa. Current management strategies consist of allergen avoidance, immunotherapy, nasal corticosteroids and systemic or topical antihistamines.

2.3.2 Cough variant asthma

Asthma is one of the most common causes of chronic cough in non-smoking adults with a normal chest radiograph and not using an ACE inhibitor; the other main causes include post-nasal drip syndrome and gastro-oesophageal reflux. In cough variant asthma, cough tends to be the predominant symptom, especially overnight and on exertion. In such individuals, lung function may be completely normal but airway hyperresponsiveness is present. The cough usually responds well to inhaled corticosteroids (ICSs).

2.3.3 Eosinophilic bronchitis

This is another condition that commonly causes chronic cough. Sputum eosinophilia is present, although typically there is no airway hyperresponsiveness, lung function is normal and no variability is present. It usually responds to ICSs.

2.3.4 Aspirin-sensitive asthma

The prevalence of aspirin-sensitive asthma is uncertain although it may exist to some extent in up to 20% of all asthmatics. Aspirin-sensitive asthma constitutes part of a syndrome where individuals demonstrate bronchoconstriction and mucosal inflammation on exposure to aspirin and other NSAIDs. Other features include nasal polyposis, rhinitis, and sometimes abdominal pain. The precise pathogenesis remains unclear, but aspirin and NSAIDs selectively inhibit cyclo-oxygenase-1, which in turn shunts arachidonic acid down the 5-lipoxygenase pathway, causing overproduction of cysteinyl leukotrienes. This has given rise to the suggestion that leukotriene receptor antagonists (LTRAs) may play a role in the management of aspirin-sensitive patients.

Patients who are sensitive to aspirin may exhibit symptoms of asthma when exposed to tartrazine. This food additive compound has a similar chemical structure to aspirin and is likely to cause symptoms in a similar way.

2.3.5 Brittle asthma

Two main clinical types of patients with brittle asthma have been described. Type I brittle asthmatics demonstrate a large and chaotic variability in PEF despite appropriate treatment. The variability has been expressed as >40% diurnal variation in PEF for >50% of the time over >150 days. Type II patients appear to have well-controlled asthma but develop unheralded severe episodes frequently requiring hospital admission. Management in both types is often difficult and affected individuals are at a greater risk of experiencing a life-threatening episode.

2.3.6 Churg–Strauss syndrome

This is a small vessel multisystem vasculitis that requires prompt recognition and appropriate management. It is a rare syndrome and is found in association with moderate to severe asthma. Other typical features include sinusitis, an eosinophil count of >1.5 x 10^9/L, pulmonary infiltrates, sinus disease, signs of a systemic vasculitis, and high serum IgE. Organ involvement is variable and it can affect the skin (purpura), nervous system (peripheral neuropathy or mononeuritis multiplex), cardiovascular system (pericarditis and heart failure), kidneys (renal failure), and gastrointestinal system (abdominal pain and bleeding). Other features such as fever, weight loss and malaise are often found. Tissue diagnosis is preferable and serum p antineutrophil cytoplasmic antibody (pANCA) is positive in about 70% of cases. Treatment consists of high dose oral corticosteroids in conjunction with immunosuppressants. The features of systemic vasculitis are often masked by patients maintained on high dose ICSs. As a result, drugs that permit a lower dose of corticosteroids, such as LTRAs, have been implicated in its development.

2.3.7 Allergic bronchopulmonary aspergillosis

This condition is caused by an immunological reaction to the fungus *Aspergillus fumigatus*. The inhalation of spores causes the appearance of eosinophilic inflammatory infiltrates in the lung. Subsequent development of fungal hyphae can cause plugging of bronchi along with bronchial wall thickening, fibrosis and bronchiectasis. Major criteria for its diagnosis are:

- A long history of asthma
- Raised peripheral blood eosinophil count (0.5–1.5 x 10^9/L)
- Fleeting chest radiographic changes such as lobar collapse (Figure 2.7) and infiltrates
- Presence of aspergillus precipitins (IgG)
- Positive RAST (or skin prick test) to *Aspergillus*
- Total serum IgE >1000 mg/ml
- Bronchiectasis.

Patients often complain of non-specific malaise, a deterioration in asthma control and cough productive of dark-coloured mucous plugs. Treatment consists of high dose corticosteroids along with antifungal pharmacotherapy, such as itraconazole, for several months (with frequent liver function test monitoring). Measuring the total IgE level is a useful tool by which to monitor treatment success.

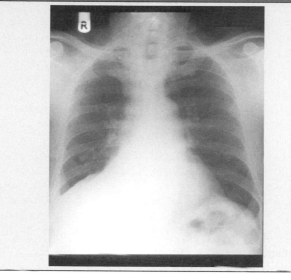

Figure 2.7 Right middle and lower lobe collapse in a patient with allergic bronchopulmonary aspergillosis

Further reading

British Guideline on the Management of Asthma (2008) British Thoracic Society Scottish Intercollegiate Guidelines Network. *Thorax* **63**(4)4: iv1–121.

Currie GP, Jackson CM, Lipworth BJ (2004) Does bronchial hyperresponsiveness matter in asthma? *Journal of Asthma* **41**: 247–58.

Smith AD, Cowan JO, Filsell S, McLachlan C, Monti-Sheehan G, Jackson P, Taylor DR (2004) Diagnosing asthma: comparisons between exhaled nitric oxide measurements and conventional tests. *Am J Respir Crit Care Med* **169**:473–8.

Taylor DR, Pijnenburg MW, Smith AD, De Jongste JC (2006) Exhaled nitric oxide measurements: clinical application and interpretation. *Thorax* **61**:817–27.

Chapter 3

Non-pharmacological management

Graeme P. Currie and John F.W. Baker

Key points

- Information about asthma (verbal and written) at a level suitable to the individual is vital
- All asthmatics should have a written, personalized action plan
- Dietary manipulation, complementary techniques, and homeopathic treatments have little or no evidence-based value in the routine management of asthma
- Smoking cessation should be encouraged in all asthmatics; a combination of behavioural strategies, nicotine replacement therapy, bupropion or varenicline can be tried.

27

International guidelines have suggested the following overall goals of asthma management:

- Prevention of troublesome symptoms of asthma during the day and night
- Prevention of exacerbations
- Maintenance of normal activity levels
- Maintenance of normal or near normal lung function
- Provision of optimal pharmacotherapy while minimizing the risk of adverse effects
- Satisfaction with the package of care provided.

Once symptoms have developed, treatment is usually indicated. This can vary from intermittent use of SABAs to combinations of oral and inhaled regimes. However, several different non-pharmacological strategies are also important in achieving goals of management.

3.1 **Asthma education programmes**

Sitting alongside appropriate pharmacological treatment, asthma education programmes are one of the main features that can contribute to its overall successful management. Such programmes should consist of:

- Written information and verbal education
- Knowledge on how to and ability to self-monitor
- Regular medical review
- Provision of an asthma action plan.

In other words, all individuals should have some understanding about their condition and be given the opportunity to find out more. They should be encouraged to regularly monitor their disease control by way of symptoms and/or PEF, and be regularly assessed by appropriately trained nursing or medical staff. Personalized, written asthma action plans play a vital role in most asthma education programmes. Moreover, every contact with a healthcare provider—whether in primary or secondary care—facilitates an opportunity to emphasize the importance of individuals being in control of their disease. Trained professionals are able to give further education, assess inhaler technique, and where necessary alter treatment. More frequent GP contacts have been shown to reduce the number of hospital admissions due to asthma and increase the length of time between these admissions.

3.2 **Asthma action plans**

Exacerbations of asthma can occur in a variety of clinical settings. Some patients experience a deterioration over a couple of days or weeks, while others develop increased symptoms upon a background of long-standing poorly controlled asthma. Written asthma action plans, tailored to the individual, provide patients with an ability to detect when asthma is becoming less well controlled and indicate what should be done about it.

Personalized asthma action plans have consistently been shown to reduce hospital admissions and attendance at accident and emergency departments. Since every individual with asthma has the potential to develop airflow obstruction, it follows that self-management plans should be incorporated into everyday routine care. Despite their documented benefit, they remain a widely under-used resource in the overall care of patients. It is important to be aware that written asthma action plans do not suit every individual. For example, some patients may require different thresholds of intervention, others may have a very individualized pharmacological regime, and those with long-standing asthma may have relatively fixed airways and little variability in PEF. However, most asthma action plans should follow a similar layout and advise:

- When to alter asthma therapy
- What to do when asthma becomes less well controlled
- How long intervention should last
- When to seek medical advice.

3.2.1 When to alter asthma therapy

Patients can be advised to alter their therapy on the basis of PEF, symptoms or a combination of these; both methods are considered to be equally effective. It is important to be aware that a reduction in PEF should be measured in relation to the individual's personal best, rather than on expected values calculated from a nomogram. This is of particular importance in those who have never achieved (or never will achieve) a predicted value or those with more fixed airflow obstruction. Table 3.1 shows a suggested relationship between PEF and symptoms according to stage of asthma control, although the clinician should be aware that modifications are often required to suit individual patients. For example, the threshold for intervention with patients with more severe asthma or previous life-threatening episodes may be lowered. This highlights the need to ensure patients are able to reliably and accurately record their own PEF measurements.

Table 3.1 Relationship between steps in asthma control according to PEF and symptoms and suggested management plans

Step	PEF	Symptoms	Management plan
1	80–100% predicted (or personal best)	Minimal or none	Continue with current treatment
2	60–80% predicted (or personal best)	Increased symptoms on exercise, at night or during a chest infection	Increase dose of ICSs
3	40–60% predicted (or personal best)	Symptoms as above plus increased SABA use with minimal relief	Start oral corticosteroids
4	<40% predicted (or personal best)	Marked symptoms, difficulty breathing	Refer to hospital

3.2.2 **What to do and how long to do it**

Current guidelines suggest that patients should double their ICS dose as the initial step when their asthma becomes less well controlled. There is no ideal length of time that such treatment should be continued. It is considered reasonable to do so for several weeks or until symptoms have resolved.

It should be noted that for some severe asthmatics, already receiving high dose ICSs, it may be reasonable to consider starting oral corticosteroids as the first line step in their asthma action plan. Despite being based on sound theoretical reasoning, there is little evidence that increasing the ICS dose outside the context of written asthma action plans is of any great benefit. However, it may well be that doing so encourages compliance and emphasizes to the patient the necessity of anti-inflammatory therapy. In patients with increased symptoms with little relief from SABAs, oral corticosteroids should be commenced. Those with more severe symptoms should call for emergency advice or be taken to hospital; oral corticosteroids and regular inhaled bronchodilators in conjunction with a period of observation might be necessary.

3.2.3 **Allergen avoidance**

The majority (but not all) of individuals with asthma display an atopic tendency. Moreover, atopic sensitization to aeroallergens may increase the likelihood of developing asthma and is associated with airway hyperresponsiveness to both direct and indirect bronchoconstrictor stimuli in those with established disease. Allergen avoidance is commonly advocated in patients with asthma, especially in those who demonstrate type 1 hypersensitivity to common aeroallergens such as house dust mite, feathers, cats and dogs. However, there is a paucity of convincing evidence-based data substantiating the effectiveness of this approach in managing asthma. For example, in a double-blind, randomized, placebo controlled study involving 1,122 individuals, the effects of house dust mite avoidance with the use of allergen-impermeable bed coverings was evaluated in terms of asthma control. Although the majority of patients in both groups were sensitized to house dust mite, avoidance was not associated with beneficial effects in lung function or other measures of asthma control. A Cochrane review has also indicated that there is little firm evidence to suggest that house dust mite avoidance measures definitely improve parameters of asthma control.

It is possible that with more complex and expensive interventions combining aeroallergen avoidance with other measures such as behavioural adaptation and environmental intervention where triggers are kept to a minimum, some benefits may occur. Similarly, there is little documented evidence to suggest that the removal of family pets such as cats or dogs is of benefit. However, such measures may well have some impact upon improving asthma symptoms in some highly atopic individuals.

3.2.4 **Dietary intervention**

All overweight patients with asthma should be advised to lose weight. This is for general health reasons and also aims to limit the degree of obesity-related breathlessness, which may be difficult to disentangle from that due to concomitant asthma. There is little convincing evidence to indicate that vitamin or mineral supplementation confers any overall significant benefit in the management of established asthma.

A number of dietary manipulation strategies have been investigated in order to assess their effect on asthma symptoms. High intakes of dietary sodium have previously been implicated in increased prevalence of asthma in the western world. Furthermore, studies have also assessed the role of sodium in bronchial hyperresponsiveness and airway inflammation. To date, results have not concluded that a diet of sodium/salt-restriction leads to a significant improvement in asthma symptoms.

The use of magnesium in acute exacerbations of asthma has led to a number of studies analyzing its use in long term management. Magnesium sulphate (unlicensed indication) given intravenously leads to improved lung function and bronchial smooth muscle relaxation in acute asthma. However, no conclusive results have been identified to recommend dietary magnesium supplementation as a long term therapy and recent guidelines have suggested a role for further study in this area.

In vitro trials have suggested the possible beneficial effects of omega 3 fatty acids in managing airways inflammation. A Cochrane review of the evidence in this field has however indicated that there is currently insufficient evidence to recommend fish oil supplementation in the management of asthma.

3.2.5 **Complementary techniques**

The Buteyko technique was developed in Russia and is a method by which individuals are encouraged to control their rate of breathing on the assumption that symptoms are due to hyperventilation and hypocapnia. Some data have suggested that it may confer some benefit in reducing breathlessness and the need for reliever treatment, but fails to influence other parameters of asthma control such as lung function. Guidelines do not advocate its use as standard treatment in the management of asthma, although it may be of some use in individuals in whom hyperventilation is a problem. There is also insufficient randomized controlled evidence to suggest that homeopathy, acupuncture or herbal preparations confer any benefit and are therefore not advised under normal circumstances. Social and environmental stressors play a significant role in asthma exacerbations. Personal relaxation and stress avoidance strategies should therefore be a key element in individualized asthma management plans.

3.2.6 **Smoking cessation**

Smoking cessation should underpin the management of all asthmatics who continue to smoke cigarettes. Not only is this important in reducing exacerbations and the prevention of smoking-related diseases, but there is also accumulating evidence that cigarette smoking reduces the efficacy of ICSs. Moreover, maternal cigarette smoking is often associated with wheeze in infants and young children. Individuals can be encouraged to stop smoking by a combination of behavioural strategies, nicotine replacement therapy and other pharmacological aids.

3.2.6.1 Behavioural support

All health professionals should encourage smokers to quit at every available opportunity; advice should be offered in an encouraging, non-judgemental and empathetic manner. It should be explained that cessation is not easy and that several attempts may be required to achieve long-term success. The following behavioural strategies may be of some use in helping individuals to succeed:

- Support a quit attempt as soon as possible, aim for total abstinence and set a date
- Review previous attempts and reflect on what has helped and what has not
- Ensure that friends and colleagues are aware that a quit attempt is planned
- Get rid of all cigarettes
- Introduce the notion that a cigarette is a killer
- Explain that cigarette smoking confers pleasure mainly because it simply prevents withdrawal symptoms
- List harmful chemicals and carcinogens that are found in cigarettes
- List diseases that cigarette smoking causes
- Discuss potential nicotine withdrawal symptoms and explain that most will pass within about a month
- Encourage patients to create goals and rewards for themselves
- Devise coping mechanisms to use during periods of craving
- Encourage partners to quit at the same time and offer them support
- Make use of follow-up support
- Use nicotine replacement therapy, bupropion or varenicline.

3.2.6.2 Nicotine replacement therapy

Nicotine replacement therapy is the most commonly used and most widely available adjunct in smoking cessation therapy. It has been shown to increase the chances of quitting by about 1.7-fold. It acts by replacing the supply of nicotine to the smoker without delivery of toxic components.

Although some forms of nicotine replacement therapy (gum, inhalator, nasal spray, lozenges) deliver nicotine more quickly than others (transdermal patches), all deliver a lower total dose, and deliver it to the brain more slowly than a cigarette. Since there is no clear evidence that any one formulation is of greater or lesser efficacy, the best approach is to follow the preference of the individual in terms of choice of product. However, in heavy smokers, the combination of a sustained release product (in order to provide continuous background nicotine) plus a more rapidly acting product for periods of craving may be of benefit. In some individuals with relative contraindications (such as acute cardiovascular disease or pregnancy) it may be prudent to use lower doses of relatively short-acting preparations. Light smokers (less than 10 cigarettes per day), or those who wait longer than an hour before their first cigarette of the day, may also be better advised to use a short-acting product in advance of their regular cigarettes or at times of craving. Treatment is generally recommended for up to 3 months, which should be followed by a gradual withdrawal. Nicotine replacement therapy is generally well tolerated, although important prescribing points are shown in Box 3.1.

Box 3.1 Important prescribing points with nicotine replacement therapy

Adverse effects

- Nausea
- Headache
- Unpleasant taste
- Hiccoughs and indigestion
- Sore throat
- Nose bleeds
- Palpitations
- Dizziness
- Insomnia
- Nasal irritation (spray).

Box 3.1 (*Contd.*)

Cautions

- Hyperthyroidism
- Diabetes mellitus
- Renal and hepatic impairment
- Gastritis and peptic ulcer disease
- Peripheral vascular disease
- Skin disorders (patches)
- Avoid nasal spray when driving or operating machinery (sneezing, watering eyes)
- Severe cardiovascular disease (arrhythmias, post-myocardial infarction)
- Recent stroke
- Pregnancy
- Breastfeeding.

3.2.6.3 Bupropion

Bupropion is of similar efficacy as nicotine replacement therapy in terms of smoking cessation rates. It is an antidepressant, although its beneficial effect upon smoking cessation is independent of this. Bupropion also helps to prevent the weight gain that is commonly associated with cessation. The main adverse effect is its association with convulsions and is therefore contraindicated in smokers with a past history of epilepsy and seizures. Bupropion should usually not be prescribed in individuals with risk factors for seizures; prescribers should also note that some drugs—such as antidepressants, antimalarials, antipsychotics, quinolones and theophylline—can lower the seizure threshold. Other important prescribing points are listed in Box 3.2. Unlike nicotine replacement therapy (which is usually started at the same time as smoking cessation), bupropion should start 1 or 2 weeks prior to the quit attempt. It should be discontinued if abstinence is not achieved within 8 weeks. There is no clear evidence that combining bupropion with nicotine replacement therapy confers any further advantage in quit rates.

3.2.6.4 Varenicline

Varenicline is a partial nicotine agonist which also blocks nicotine receptors from stimulation by free nicotine. It is an effective smoking cessation oral drug which increases the likelihood of quitting by a factor of about 2.3, and is therefore slightly more effective than nicotine replacement therapy or bupropion. There is no evidence that combining varenicline with other therapies is any more effective than varenicline alone. Varenicline should be started 1–2 weeks prior to the planned quit day, with increasing doses over the first

> **Box 3.2 Contraindications to prescribing bupropion**
>
> - History of seizures
> - Use of drugs that lower the seizure threshold
> - Alcohol or benzodiazepine withdrawal
> - Eating disorders
> - Bipolar illness
> - Central nervous system tumours
> - Pregnancy and breastfeeding
> - Hepatic cirrhosis

few days and continued for 12 weeks in total. The most common side effect of varenicline is nausea.

Both varenicline and bupropion have been implicated in cases of depression and suicidal ideation. Consequently, the US Food and Drug Administration require both of these products to carry a "black box" safety warning due to the potential risks of depression, suicidal thoughts and suicidal actions.

Further reading

Cahill K, Stead LF, Lancaster T. (2008) Nicotine receptor partial agonists for smoking cessation. *Cochrane Database of Systematic Reviews* Issue 3. Art. No.: CD006103. DOI: 10.1002/14651858.CD006103.pub3.

Cooper S, Osborne J, Newton S, et al. (2003) Effect of two breathing exercises (Buteyko and pranayama) in asthma: a randomised controlled trial. *Thorax* **58**: 674–9.

Gøtzsche PC, Johansen HK, Schmidt LM, Burr ML. (2004) House dust mite control measures for asthma. *Cochrane Database of Systematic Reviews*, 2004. CD001187.

Gibson PG, Powell H. (2004) Written action plans for asthma: an evidence-based review of the key components. *Thorax* **59**: 94–9.

Hughes JR, Stead LF, Lancaster T (2007) Antidepressants for smoking cessation. *Cochrane Database of Systematic Reviews* Issue 1. Art. No.: CD000031. DOI: 10.1002/14651858.CD000031.pub3.

Morgan WJ, Crain EF, Gruchalla RS, et al. (2004) Results of a home-based environmental intervention among urban children with asthma. *N Engl J Med* **351**: 1068–80.

Srivastava PS, Currie GP, Britton J. (2006) ABC of chronic obstructive pulmonary disease: smoking cessation. *Br Med J* **332**: 1324–6.

Stead LF, Perera R, Bullen C, Mant D, Lancaster T (2008) Nicotine replacement therapy for smoking cessation. *Cochrane Database of Systematic Reviews* Issue 1. Art. No.: CD000146. DOI: 10.1002/14651858.CD000146.pub3.

Woodcock A, Forster L, Matthews E, et al. (2003) Control of exposure to mite allergen and allergen-impermeable bed covers for adults with asthma. *N Engl J Med* **349**: 225–36.

Chapter 4

Pharmacological management

Graeme P. Currie

Key points

- UK guidelines advocate five steps in the pharmacological management of asthma in adults
- The overall aims are to establish early control, maintain control and step down treatment following 3–6 months of clinical stability
- Prior to escalating treatment, patients should have good concordance, have a satisfactory inhaler technique, and not be exposed to trigger factors wherever possible
- SABAs should be used on an 'as required' basis in most asthmatics (step 1).
- Regular low to moderate doses of ICSs are required (step 2):
  - When SABAs are used > several times per week
  - When symptoms are present > twice per week
  - When patients wake overnight due to asthma
  - Following a recent exacerbation
- In patients with persistent symptoms, frequent reliever use and exacerbations despite an adequate dose of ICS, a long-acting β_2-agonist (LABA) should be added (step 3)
- Further options include the addition of a LTRA, theophylline or a higher ICS dose (step 4)
- In a minority of persistent asthmatics receiving step 4 treatment, regular use of low dose oral steroid should be considered (step 5).

4.1 **Pharmacological management of asthma**

4.1.1 **Overview**

The British Thoracic Society guidelines suggest that chronic adult asthma should be managed in a stepwise fashion (Figure 4.1). Treatment can be started at any of the five steps—largely determined by severity of symptoms—in an attempt to rapidly control symptoms. Before escalating treatment thereafter, clinicians should firstly determine that:

- The inhaler device is being used correctly
- Treatment is being adhered to
- Individuals are not being unnecessarily exposed to triggers.

Once symptoms have been stable for a 3–6-month period, therapy should usually be back titrated. This means that patients are maintained on the minimum amount of treatment that satisfactorily controls symptoms.

4.1.1.1 Assessment of asthma control

There is no perfect tool by which to assess asthma control, although this is an integral facet of overall asthma management. In everyday practice, it is usually assessed by determining:

- Frequency of reliever use
- Frequency of wheeze and chest tightness
- Frequency of nocturnal symptoms
- Limitation of activity due to symptoms of asthma
- Variation in PEF
- Frequency of exacerbations.
- FEV_1

Various questionnaires have been developed to help assess degree of asthma control. These include the asthma control test, asthma control questionnaire and asthma therapy assessment questionnaire. Such patient-centred questionnaires generally involve determining limitation to daily activities, degree of breathlessness and wheezing, sleep disturbance, use of relief inhalers, lung function and overall asthma control.

In recent years, there has been interest in non-invasive tools by which to measure the extent of underlying inflammation with the potential aim of titrating anti-inflammatory treatment to optimum levels, improving asthma control and minimizing adverse effects. The most widely used biomarkers used in this respect include exhaled nitric oxide, sputum eosinophils, and airway hyperresponsiveness to different bronchoconstrictor stimuli. All of these tools have their benefits and drawbacks. In the future, measuring a surrogate inflammatory biomarker such as exhaled nitric oxide may become the norm before deciding when to alter the ICS dose or adding in a further second line agent (Table 4.1).

Table 4.1 Characteristic features of the ideal surrogate inflammatory biomarker by which to monitor the response to treatment and subsequently titrate therapy
Raised only in asthma
Raised only when endobronchial inflammation is presen
Portable
Inexpensive
Easy to measure in primary and secondary care settings
Acceptable to patients
Linear reduction on institution of anti-inflammatory therapy with a demonstrable clear cut dose-response effect
Demonstrated to provide better clinical control when used along with conventional measures than with the latter alone

Figure 4.1 Stepwise management of chronic asthma in adults

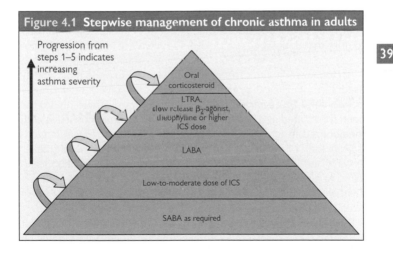

Progression from steps 1–5 indicates increasing asthma severity

Oral corticosteroid

LTRA, slow release β₂-agonist, theophylline or higher ICS dose

LABA

Low-to-moderate dose of ICS

SABA as required

4.1.2 **Step 1: SABAs**

SABAs such as salbutamol and terbutaline act directly upon bronchial smooth muscle β_2-adrenoceptors and cause the airways to dilate for up to 4–6 hours. These drugs are very quick acting, and patients can often perceive effects within 5–10 minutes of use.

All patients with asthma should be advised to use their short-acting β_2-agonist on an 'as required' basis; no additional benefit is conferred by regular use.

There is no clear threshold at which patients should move to step 2, but it is reasonable to initiate regular anti-inflammatory therapy if patients are using their SABA more than several times a week. Other suggested thresholds include an exacerbation of asthma in the preceding 2 years, symptoms of active asthma > twice a week and waking overnight at least once a week due to asthma.

4.1.3 **Step 2: ICSs**

ICSs are a vital component in the successful treatment of persistent asthma of most severities. Of all treatment in the long-term control of asthma, ICSs are by far the most potent, effective and widely studied class of drug. Once bound to cytoplasmic receptors concentrated in airway epithelial and endothelial cells, they increase and decrease the gene transcription of anti-inflammatory and proinflammatory mediators, respectively. Corticosteroids also exert a direct inhibitory effect upon a number of cells (eosinophils, T lymphocytes, epithelial cells) implicated in the asthmatic inflammatory process and attenuate airway hyperresponsiveness. Over time, they cause the airways to dilate.

The starting dose of ICSs should be decided according to the severity of symptoms. This is normally between 400 and 800 micrograms/day of beclometasone or equivalent in adults. It is important to note that fluticasone and ciclesonide are twice as potent as beclometasone and budesonide on a microgram equivalent basis.

Beclometasone, fluticasone, and budesonide are the most widely used ICSs in clinical practice, although a relatively new drug—ciclesonide—represents a major step forward. Ciclesonide has been formulated as a pro-drug meaning that it remains inactive until metabolized in lung tissue to its active compound (desisobutyryl-ciclesonide). Moreover, it has been developed to reach the smaller airways and is delivered by way of the propellant hydrofluouroalkane. As a consequence, the lung deposition of ciclesonde is approximately 50% of the delivered dose, with only 1% of the drug freely circulating (Figure 4.2).

Dose-response studies using ICSs have demonstrated that most therapeutic gain is achieved with beclometasone equivalent doses up to 800 micrograms/day; at doses above this, there is an exponential increase in adverse effects with little further gain in terms of lung function (Figure 4.3). In other words, at daily doses of >800 micrograms of beclometasone or equivalent in adults, the dose–response curve for desired effects becomes flat, while that for systemic adverse effects becomes steep. However, due to the heterogeneity of asthma, it is likely that some patients do experience further benefit in asthma control with higher doses. Indeed, in patients with persistent symptoms

Figure 4.2 Pharmacologic characteristics of ciclesonide and its active metabolite desisobutyryl-ciclesonide

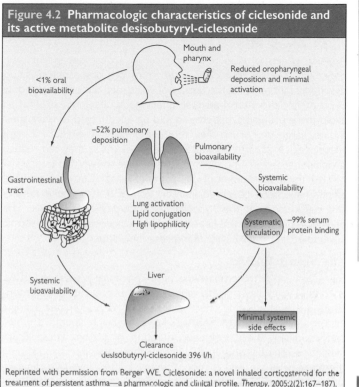

Mouth and pharynx

Reduced oropharyngeal deposition and minimal activation

<1% oral bioavailability

−52% pulmonary deposition

Pulmonary bioavailability

Systemic bioavailability

Gastrointestinal tract

Lung activation
Lipid conjugation
High lipophilicity

Systematic circulation

−99% serum protein binding

Systemic bioavailability

Liver

Minimal systemic side effects

Clearance desisobutyryl-ciclesonide 396 l/h

Reprinted with permission from Berger WE. Ciclesonide: a novel inhaled corticosteroid for the treatment of persistent asthma—a pharmacologic and clinical profile. *Therapy*. 2005;2(2):167–187.

Figure 4.3 Dose-response curve effect of ICSs in asthma

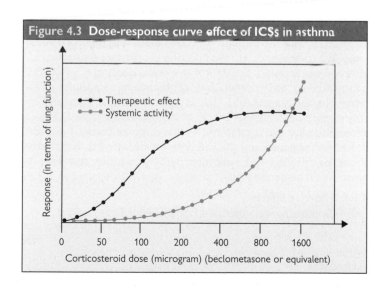

Response (in terms of lung function)

- Therapeutic effect
- Systemic activity

0   50   100   200   400   800   1600

Corticosteroid dose (microgram) (beclometasone or equivalent)

despite using 800 micrograms/day of ICS plus a LABA, one therapeutic option (step 4) is to further increase the dose of ICS.

4.1.3.1 Adverse effects

Adverse effects of ICSs tend to occur in a dose-dependant way. However, at doses up to 800 micrograms/day, oral candidiasis and dysphonia (alteration in the quality of voice) are the only commonly encountered short-term adverse effects in adults. In an attempt to avoid these problems, patients should be encouraged to rinse their mouth, gargle and brush their teeth after taking their ICS. Using a spacer device can also minimize these problems as they can reduce oropharyngeal deposition. Some studies have shown that skin bruising occurs more commonly in patients using ICSs, and variable effects have been observed in reduction of bone mineral density and suppression of the hypothalamic–pituitary–adrenal axis. The once daily ICS ciclesonide has been shown to have little or no systemic adverse effects at far higher than prescribed doses.

4.1.4 **Step 3: LABAs**

Salmeterol and formoterol are the most commonly prescribed LABAs. Both bind to airway smooth muscle β_2-adrenoceptors and demonstrate a bronchodilating effect in excess of 12 hours after a single inhalation. In contrast to SABAs, LABAs are highly lipophilic, which partly explains their prolonged duration of action. These drugs exhibit no clinically meaningful anti-inflammatory effects and should therefore *never* be used as monotherapy. LABAs have two clinically important properties, namely a bronchodilator effect in the presence of low bronchomotor tone and a protective effect in the presence of increased bronchomotor tone.

Various studies have shown that the addition of a LABA is usually superior to doubling the dose of ICS in those with persistent symptoms. As a consequence, in individuals who experience persistent symptoms and exacerbations despite low-to-medium doses of ICS (400–800 micrograms/day of beclometasone or equivalent), guidelines advocate a therapeutic trial of LABA as add on therapy. If there is no clinical response, the LABA should be discontinued and the ICS dose increased to 800 micrograms/day. If some response occurs, the LABA should be continued and the ICS dose be increased to 800 micrograms/day (Figure 4.4). If symptoms persist thereafter, step 4 treatment should be considered.

4.1.4.1 Adverse effects

LABAs are usually well tolerated, but adverse effects include:

- Tachycardia
- Fine tremour
- Headache
- Muscle cramps

- Prolongation of the QT interval
- Hypokalaemia
- Feelings of nervousness.

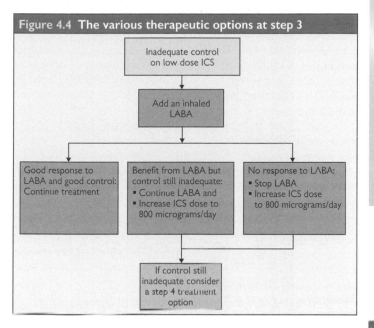

Figure 4.4 **The various therapeutic options at step 3**

Several studies have suggested that long-term use of a LABA (salmeterol) may be associated with an increase in asthma-related deaths and life threatening events in susceptible populations such as African Americans. However, these findings may have been due to the fact that many of the individuals included in the clinical trials were using LABAs as monotherapy (without regular anti-inflammatory treatment). Nevertheless, this prompted the United States Food and Drug Administration to announce important safety information regarding inhalers containing LABAs and to advise that new labelling be produced outlining the 'small but significant risk in asthma-related deaths' associated with their regular use.

4.1.4.2 Combined ICS plus LABA inhalers
The use of an ICS combined with a LABA in a single device is becoming an increasingly popular method of delivering two drugs to the lung (Table 4.2). In asthmatics with persistent symptoms despite adequate doses of ICSs, commonsense suggests that such an approach would appear to be a reasonable to consider. Moreover, this is the logical pharmacological option since ICSs are the most potent anti-inflammatory agents and LABAs are the most potent

Table 4.2 Constituents and adult dosing regimes of Seretide, Symbicort® and Fostair

Brand name	ICS	LABA	Inhaler device	Dose ICS/LABA (micrograms)	Number of puffs (twice daily)
Seretide®	Fluticasone	Salmeterol	Evohaler	50/25 125/25 250/25	2 2 2
Seretide®	Fluticasone	Salmeterol	Accuhaler	100/50 250/50 500/50	1 1
Symbicort®	Budesonide	Formoterol	Turbohaler	100/6 200/6	1–2 1–2
Fostair®	Beclometasone	Formoterol	MDI	100/6	1–2

bronchodilators available. Currently, salmeterol can be given with fluticasone in a single inhaler (Seretide®) and formoterol can be given with either budesonide (Symbicort®) or beclometasone (Fostair®) in a single inhaler; other combinations of ICSs plus LABAs in a single inhaler are in varying stages of development. Fostair® is the most recently introduced combination inhaler and the only such inhaler that contains extra fine particles which are deposited into the smaller airways within the lungs.

Possible advantages of combination inhalers include:

- Fewer inhalations
- Fewer inhaler devices
- Patients perceive fairly immediate bronchodilatation due to the LABA moiety (especially with combination inhalers containing formoterol which has an onset of action similar to salbutamol)
- Anti-inflammatory concordance is facilitated due to the inseparable nature of the inhaler constituents
- Potential synergistic action between the ICSs and LABAs when given together.

Possible disadvantages of combination inhalers include:

- Altering the ICS dose (without altering the LABA dose) is less straightforward
- Patients may be started on combination inhalers as first line preventer treatment rather than ICSs alone (in other words temptation may result in step 3 treatment being initiated when step 2 treatment would be perfectly adequate)
- Relative expense
- More difficulty in back-titrating treatment without the provision of a separate inhaler device containing ICS alone.

4.1.4.3 Symbicort® "SMART" regime

In adult patients with poorly controlled asthma at step 3, studies have shown that using Symbicort® 200/6 on both a regular (twice daily) basis along with the same inhaler for as required use (instead of a SABA) can result in better control of asthma: this is the so-called SMART (**S**ingle **M**aintenance **A**nd **R**eliever **T**herapy) method. Such an approach has mainly been shown to be effective in exacerbation reduction, as a consequence of delivery of anti-inflammatory treatment to the airways during periods of heightened inflammation (i.e. symptoms of asthma) along with the fairly immediate "bronchodilator boost" facilitated by formoterol. Published data indicate that the SMART approach does not generally result in patients overusing Symbicort®, although they are advised to seek medical help if >8 puffs are used daily.

4.1.5 **Step 4: LTRAs**

Cysteinyl leukotrienes (C_4, D_4 and E_4)—previously known as the slow relaxing substance of anaphylaxis—are lipid mediators produced from arachidonic acid (Figure 4.5). Following synthesis, cysteinyl leukotrienes activate cell membrane receptors found on airway smooth muscle and macrophages. This results in a variety of undesirable effects in the airway such as:

- Mucous hypersecretion
- Hypertrophy and proliferation of smooth muscle
- Bronchoconstriction
- Inhibition of mucociliary clearance
- Increased pulmonary vascular permeability
- Recruitment of inflammatory cells
- Release of acetylcholine from nerve fibres.

The effects of cysteinyl leukotrienes in the airway can be influenced by inhibiting their formation (using a 5-lipoxygenase inhibitor) or more commonly by preventing binding to their receptor (using a LTRA). Zileuton (not licensed for use in the UK) is the only licensed 5-lipoxygenase inhibitor and is available for use in only some countries; regular treatment necessitates frequent liver function tests to monitor for potential hepatotoxicity. Montelukast, zafirlukast (Figure 4.6 and Table 4.3) and pranlukast (pranlukast is not licensed for use in the UK) are orally active LTRAs that selectively antagonize the cell surface cysteinyl leukotriene 1 receptor. These drugs confer both weak anti-inflammatory and bronchodilator effects; they also attenuate airway hyperresponsiveness (Table 4.3).

Current guidelines suggest that a LTRA should be considered when either the combination of an inhaled corticosteroid plus LABA fails to satisfactorily control symptoms, or following a failed trial of LABA (step 4). LTRAs may also have some use in:

- Patients with both asthma and allergic rhinitis
- Exercise-induced asthma
- Aspirin-induced asthma
- Asthmatics who are unable or unwilling to use inhaler devices.

4.1.5.1 Adverse effects

LTRAs are generally well tolerated. However, adverse effects such as hypersensitivity reactions, arthralgia, pulmonary eosinophilia, gastrointestinal disturbances, sleep disorders, respiratory infections, hallucinations, seizures, and raised liver enzymes have been reported. In the UK, LTRAs are not advised in pregnancy unless absolutely essential. Concern has been raised regarding the development of Churg–Strauss syndrome and administration of leukotriene receptor antagonists, although many of the documented cases have

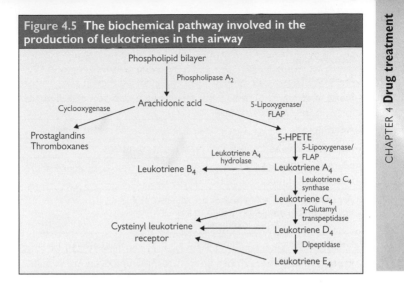

Figure 4.5 The biochemical pathway involved in the production of leukotrienes in the airway

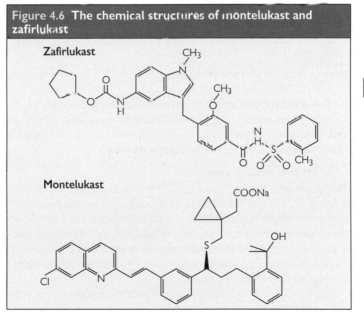

Figure 4.6 The chemical structures of montelukast and zafirlukast

Table 4.3 Prescribing and pharmacokinetic data for montelukast and zafirlukast

Generic name	Montelukast	Zafirlukast
Brand name	Singulair®	Accolate®
Mode of action	Inhibitor of leukotriene receptor	Inhibitor of leukotriene receptor
Adult dose	10 mg daily	20 mg twice daily
Paediatric licence	Yes	No
Prescribing in renal impairment	No dose adjustment	No dose adjustment
Prescribing in hepatic impairment	No dose adjustment in mild to moderate dysfunction	Reduced clearance
Use in pregnancy	Limited data	Limited data
Protein binding	>99%	>99%
Half-life	2.7–5.5 hours	10 hours
Time to peak levels	3–4 hours	3 hours
Bioavailability	64%	Uncertain
Special instructions	Can be taken with food	Avoid with food
Interaction with warfarin	Not known to interact	Increases prothrombin time

occurred where concomitant leukotriene receptor antagonist has allowed a reduction in ICS dose. This in turn suggests that latent Churg–Strauss syndrome may have been unmasked by a decrease in anti-inflammatory therapy delivered to the lungs.

4.1.6 **Step 4: methylxanthines**

Theophylline is the most common methylxanthine used in the treatment of asthma and has a chemical structure (and some properties) similar to caffeine (Figure 4.7). It is a phosphodiesterase inhibitor and demonstrates activity in a multitude of cell types throughout the body. It also has a variety of other effects such as increased interleukin-10 release, enhanced apoptosis, inflammatory mediator inhibition and increased catecholamine release.

Despite its modest clinical efficacy in asthma, theophylline is orally active and relatively inexpensive, in turn making it an attractive therapeutic option, especially in less wealthy populations. When used in asthma, these drugs confer weak bronchodilator and anti-inflammatory effects. Current guidelines suggest that a therapeutic trial of theophylline can be considered in patients with persistent symptoms despite a low-to-moderate dose of ICS plus LABA (step 4). Theophyllines

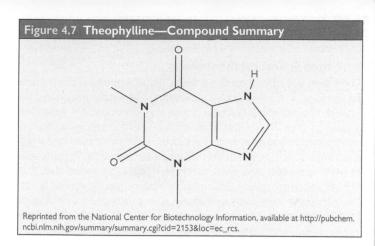

Figure 4.7 Theophylline—Compound Summary

Reprinted from the National Center for Biotechnology Information, available at http://pubchem.
ncbi.nlm.nih.gov/summary/summary.cgi?cid=2153&loc=ec_rcs.

should initially be started at a low to moderate dose and the plasma concentration checked before titrating the dose upwards, or when adding in a new drug which may alter its metabolism. Target levels are between 10 and 20 mg/L (55–110 µM). At theophylline concentrations greater than this, the frequency of adverse effects may increase to unacceptable levels.

4.1.6.1 Adverse effects
The use of theophylline is frequently limited due to concerns of cardiac arrhythmias, gastrointestinal upset, and the need for monitoring plasma levels due to a narrow therapeutic index. Moreover, there is considerable variation in the half-life of theophylline and care needs to be taken in certain medical conditions and when using particular drugs that alter its half-life and plasma clearance.

Causes of increased plasma theophylline levels (i.e. reduced plasma clearance) include:

- Heart failure
- Liver cirrhosis
- Advanced age
- Ciprofloxacin
- Erythromycin
- Clarithromycin
- Verapamil
- Causes of reduced plasma theophylline levels (i.e. increased plasma clearance) include:
  - cigarette smoking
  - alcoholism
  - rifampicin
  - phenytoin

- carbamazepine
- lithium.

4.1.7 **Step 5: oral corticosteroids**

Long-term use of oral corticosteroids (usually prednisolone) should be avoided if at all possible, although if absolutely necessary, the lowest possible dose (such as 5 mg/day) that controls symptoms should be used (Figure 4.8). They should only be used under specialist supervision and an attempt to discontinue them should be considered after 3 months and at regular intervals thereafter. Patients who receive long-term oral corticosteroids should be aware that they should not be stopped suddenly and a slow reduction in dose is usually necessary. Immediate withdrawal after prolonged administration may lead to acute adrenal insufficiency and even death; all patients receiving oral corticosteroids should be given a treatment card alerting others on the problems associated with abrupt discontinuation. Courses of oral corticosteroids that last less than 3 weeks do not normally require to be tapered before stopping.

4.1.7.1 Adverse effects

The risk of corticosteroid-induced osteoporosis is related to cumulative dose. This implies that in addition to individuals on maintenance prednisolone, those requiring frequent courses may experience long-term complications. Patients using at least 7.5 mg/day of prednisolone (or equivalent) for 3 months are at heightened risk of adverse effects along with those over the age of 65 years. Prolonged use of oral corticosteroids can be associated with a variety of other undesirable adverse effects. Examples of these are shown in Figure 4.9.

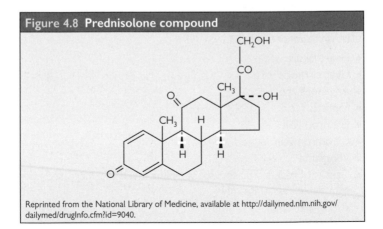

Figure 4.8 Prednisolone compound

Reprinted from the National Library of Medicine, available at http://dailymed.nlm.nih.gov/dailymed/drugInfo.cfm?id=9040.

4.1.8 **Other drugs and approaches**

4.1.8.1 Anti-immunoglobulin E

Many individuals with asthma are atopic, with the consequence that aeroallergens interact with immunoglobulin E (IgE) and cause the release of inflammatory mediators. Humanized recombinant monoclonal anti-IgE molecules have been developed for the treatment of IgE-mediated disease processes such as asthma; these drugs attenuate the activity of IgE by linking to the constant region of the IgE molecule. This in turn prevents circulating IgE from interacting with receptors on a variety of inflammatory cells (Figure 4.10).

The most widely used anti-IgE drug is omalizumab; it has been shown to reduce symptoms, reduce exacerbation frequency, improve quality of life, and facilitate a reduction in ICS dose. It has also been shown to have beneficial effects in patients with asthma and concomitant allergic rhinitis. Omalizumab is given as a sub-cutaneous injection every 2–4 weeks, with the dose and frequency being determined by baseline IgE levels and body weight; it is not licensed for use in patients with IgE levels >1500 IU/l. It should only be given under specialist advice in centres experienced in dealing with patients with difficult asthma. Although it is well tolerated, adverse effects such as anaphylaxis (even after a year of treatment) and skin reactions have been reported.

Omalizumab is licensed for use in adults who have severe persistent allergic asthma despite high dose ICSs and LABAs with impaired lung function and frequent exacerbations. In particular, the UK National Institute for Health and Clinical Excellence advises that omalizumab should be considered only for patients who have had at least two severe exacerbations requiring hospital admission within the previous year, whereas the Scottish Medicines Consortium advises its restriction to patients requiring maintenance oral steroids when all other treatments have failed.

4.1.8.2 Macrolides

Macrolide antibiotics—such as clarithromycin—exhibit a degree of anti-inflammatory activity. As a result, they are sometimes given to patients in a low daily dose under specialist supervision.

4.1.8.3 Anti-cholinergics

Short and long acting anti-cholinergics have no role in the long term management of asthma. Tiotropium is widely used in COPD, and although it may confer some benefit in patients with chronic asthma with fixed airflow obstruction (and thereby exhibit some properties of COPD), it is not licensed for this purpose.

4.1.8.4 Immunosuppressants

In the most severe asthmatics who require high doses of oral corticosteroids for prolonged periods of time, immunosuppressants may

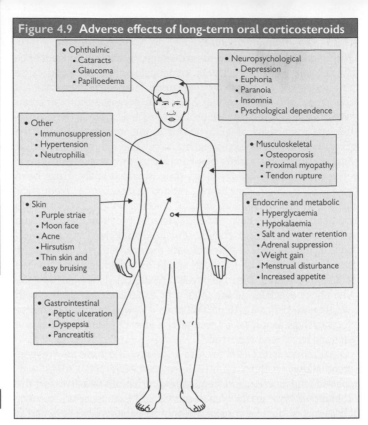

Figure 4.9 Adverse effects of long-term oral corticosteroids

- Ophthalmic
  - Cataracts
  - Glaucoma
  - Papilloedema

- Neuropsychological
  - Depression
  - Euphoria
  - Paranoia
  - Insomnia
  - Pyschological dependence

- Other
  - Immunosuppression
  - Hypertension
  - Neutrophilia

- Musculoskeletal
  - Osteoporosis
  - Proximal myopathy
  - Tendon rupture

- Skin
  - Purple striae
  - Moon face
  - Acne
  - Hirsutism
  - Thin skin and easy bruising

- Endocrine and metabolic
  - Hyperglycaemia
  - Hypokalaemia
  - Salt and water retention
  - Adrenal suppression
  - Weight gain
  - Menstrual disturbance
  - Increased appetite

- Gastrointestinal
  - Peptic ulceration
  - Dyspepsia
  - Pancreatitis

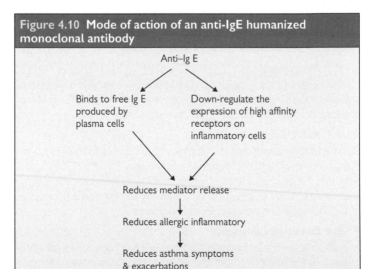

Figure 4.10 Mode of action of an anti-IgE humanized monoclonal antibody

Anti–Ig E

Binds to free Ig E produced by plasma cells

Down-regulate the expression of high affinity receptors on inflammatory cells

Reduces mediator release

Reduces allergic inflammatory

Reduces asthma symptoms & exacerbations

be occasionally tried under expert supervision; examples of these include methotrexate, ciclosporin and gold. The potential risks and benefits of these agents should be fully discussed with patients before a 3–6 month trial is considered.

4.1.8.5 Bronchial thermoplasty

An increase in airway smooth muscle mass is often found in asthmatics, and is considered to be an important factor in those with severe or fatal asthma. Bronchial thermoplasty is a novel treatment still undergoing evaluation, where controlled thermal energy is delivered to the airway wall during several bronchoscopy procedures. This in turn results in a prolonged reduction of airway smooth muscle mass. In individuals with moderate to severe asthma, bronchial thermoplasty has been shown to confer some benefit in reducing symptoms, reliever use and exacerbations and in improving quality of life and lung function. Further large, long-term studies are required to fully evaluate this new procedure and determine which patients may benefit most.

Further reading

Barnes PJ (2007) Using a combination inhaler (budesonide plus formoterol) as rescue therapy improves asthma control. *BMJ* **335**: 513.

Bateman ED, Boushey HA, Bousquet J, et al. (2004) Can guideline-defined asthma control be achieved? The Gaining Optimal Asthma Control study. *Am J Respir Crit Care Med* **170**: 836–44.

Currie GP, McLaughlin K. (2006) The expanding role of leukotriene receptor antagonists in chronic asthma. *Ann Allergy Asthma Immunol* **97**: 731–42.

Gentile DA, Skoner DP (2010) New asthma drugs: small molecule inhaled corticosteroids. *Curr Opin Pharmacol* **10**: 260–5.

Masoli M, Weatherall M, Holt S, et al. (2005) Moderate dose inhaled corticosteroids plus salmeterol versus higher doses of inhaled corticosteroids in symptomatic asthma. *Thorax* **60**: 730–4.

Nelson HS, Weiss ST, Bleecker ER, Yancey SW, Dorinsky PM (2006) The Salmeterol Multicenter Asthma Research Trial: a comparison of usual pharmacotherapy for asthma or usual pharmacotherapy plus salmeterol. *Chest* **129**: 15–26.

Peters SP, Kunselman SJ, Icitovic N, Moore WC, Pascual R, Ameredes BT, Boushey HA, Calhoun WJ, Castro M, Cherniack RM, Craig T, Denlinger L, Engle LL, DiMango EA, Fahy JV, Israel E, Jarjour N, Kazani SD, Kraft M, Lazarus SC, Lemanske RF Jr, Lugogo N, Martin RJ, Meyers DA, Ramsdell J, Sorkness CA, Sutherland ER, Szefler SJ, Wasserman SI, Walter MJ, Wechsler ME, Chinchilli VM, Bleecker ER Tiotropium bromide step-up therapy for adults with uncontrolled asthma. (2010) National Heart, Lung, and Blood Institute Asthma Clinical Research Network. *N Engl J Med*; **363**: 1715–26.

Postma DS, O'Byrne PM, Pedersen S (2011) Comparison of the effect of low-dose ciclesonide and fixed-dose fluticasone propionate and salmeterol combination on long-term asthma control. *Chest* **139**: 311–18.

Shrewsbury S, Pyke S, Britton M. (2000) Meta-analysis of increased dose of inhaled corticosteroid or addition of salmeterol in symptomatic asthma (MIASMA). *Br Med J* **320**: 1368–73.

Walker S, Monteil M, Phelan K, Lasserson TJ, Walters EH. Anti-IgE for chronic asthma in adults and children. *Cochrane Database of Systematic Reviews* 2006, Issue 2. Art. No. CD003559. DOI: 10.1002/14651858.CD003559.pub3.

Chapter 5

Inhalers

Graeme P. Currie

Key Points

- Correct inhaler technique is an integral component in the management of asthma and should be assessed at every available opportunity as technique often declines over time
- Patients should be given specific instructions on use of the particular inhaler and be able to use it with confidence
- Dry powder inhalers (DPIs) reduce the need for co-ordination and are easier to use than pressurized metered dose inhalers (pMDIs)
- Spacer devices help overcome problems with co-ordination encountered with metered dose inhalers (MDIs) and reduce pharyngeal deposition
- If a patient is unable to use a particular device, an alternative should be considered.

5.1 **Inhalers**

Drugs have been administered by inhalation for thousands of years. For example, between 2000–1500 BC in Egypt and India, herbal preparations were burned and the vapours inhaled. Over subsequent years, a variety of medicinal and non-medicinal substances have been inhaled as treatments for breathlessness, and eventually a primitive nebulizer was developed in the mid-1800s. In 1929, the potential benefits of inhaled adrenaline were reported for patients with obstructive lung disorders and pMDIs were introduced in the 1950s.

Most drugs used in asthma are inhaled through the mouth using hand-held devices. This makes intuitive sense as these drugs are then delivered topically to the airways in an attempt to overcome airway obstruction and attenuate inflammation. Unfortunately, only a small proportion of drug reaches the lungs, as a considerable amount is deposited in the mouth, throat and vocal cords and subsequently swallowed (Figure 5.1). This problem is accentuated with pMDI, as difficulties are often encountered with co-ordinating actuation and inhalation. Further issues leading to sub-optimal delivery are found in older patients, while concordance (in both "real-life" and clinical studies) with most inhaled devices, is often sub-optimal. It is important that assessment and correction of inhaler technique is carried out at every available opportunity, as over time patients often become less able to use their inhaler correctly. Moreover, an increasingly bewildering array of inhaler devices is now available and problems often arise for both the clinician and patient as to which type should be prescribed. Many advantages and disadvantages of different inhaler types exist (Table 5.1); no perfect inhaler exists, but desirable attributes are shown in Box 5.1.

Figure 5.1 Only a small amount of the drug leaving a MDI reaches the lungs

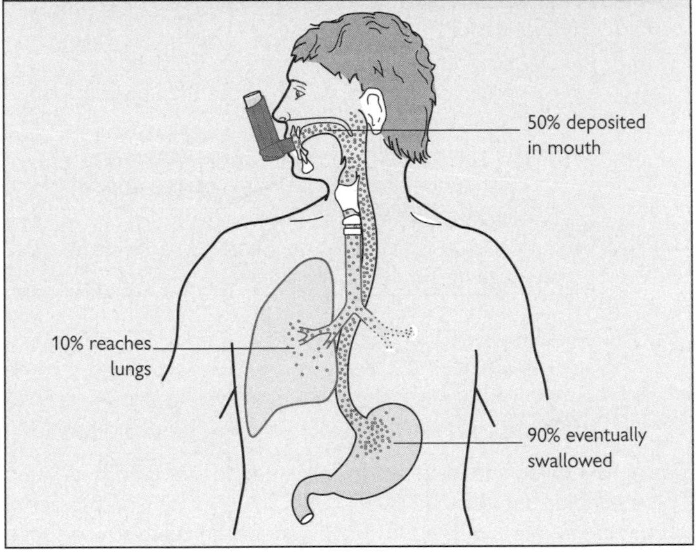

50% deposited in mouth

10% reaches lungs

90% eventually swallowed

Table 5.1 Advantages and disadvantages of different types of inhaler devices in asthma

Type of inhaler	Advantages	Disadvantages
MDI	Portable Inexpensive Can be used quickly Short treatment time Contain high numbers of doses	Actuation and inhalation co-ordination required Cold freon effect High potential for poor technique Usually no dose counter
MDI with spacer	More effective drug delivery Reduced oropharyngeal drug deposition No cold freon effect Useful in emergency situations	Bulky Maintenance/priming required to overcome electrostatic charges Less portable Education required for correct use Additional cost of spacer Usually no dose counter
DPIs (Turbohaler® and Accuhaler®)	No actuation/inhalation co-ordination necessary Portable May have a dose counter Spacer unnecessary Short treatment time	Adequate inspiratory flow required More expensive than pMDIs No propellant Should not be stored in damp environments
Breath activated MDIs (Easi-Breathe® and autohaler)	No actuation/inhalation co-ordination necessary Portable Short treatment time	Cold freon effect Adequate inspiratory flow required
Nebulizer	Tidal breathing adequate Easy to use Patient preference	Less portable, noisy and indiscreet Expensive and maintenance required Unpredictable lung deposition Variable performance Drug wastage Long drug delivery time Need for a power source

> **Box 5.1 Attributes of the ideal inhaler**
>
> - Ease of use during an acute episode of breathlessness
> - Ease of use as maintenance treatment
> - Easy to learn how to use
> - Quick delivery of drug
> - Portable, lightweight, hygienic and discreet
> - Moisture resistant
> - Same type of inhaler for different drugs
> - Ability to tell that a dose has been taken
> - A dose counter to reflect how many inhalations remain
> - No unpleasant local effects/taste
> - Effective delivery of drug to the endobronchial tree
> - Inexpensive
> - Harmless to the environment
> - Easily refillable
> - Little or no maintenance or cleaning required.

In practice, when prescribing an inhaler, the over-riding principles should be a combination of:

- Ensuring the patient can use the device correctly and consistently
- Providing adequate instruction given by someone skilled in doing so
- Switching to an alternative and more suitable device if necessary
- Patient preference
- Ease and practicality of use.

5.2 **Types of inhalers**

5.2.1 **MDIs**

The most common inhaler device is a pMDI (Figure 5.2) which can deliver SABAs, LABAs, ICSs, and LABAs plus ICSs in combination. Patients however often have difficulty in using pMDIs, particularly co-ordinating actuation of the device with an adequate inspiratory effort. Other common errors in pMDI use includes failure to exhale before actuation, too short a breath-hold following inspiration, and too rapid an inspiratory flow. Moreover, radiolabelled studies have shown that only around 10% of the emitted drug—even with good technique—reaches the lungs. To correctly use a pMDI, patients should carry out the following steps:

- Remove the mouthpiece cover (if there is one) and shake the inhaler

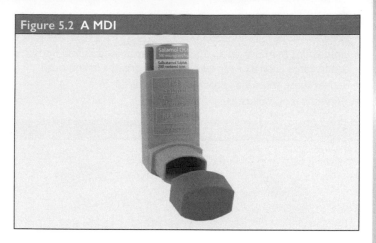

Figure 5.2 A MDI

- Breathe out fully
- Put your lips firmly around the mouthpiece
- Press only once with the inhaler in the mouth and at the same time breathe inwards fully and deeply
- Hold your breath for up to 10 seconds or as long as you find comfortable
- Breathe out normally
- Repeat these steps if a second puff is required
- Wipe the mouthpiece clean and replace its protective cover.

Some patients develop oropharyngeal candidiasis and complain of an alteration in the voice quality (dysphonia) when using a pMDI to deliver inhaled steroids. The risk of developing these problems can be minimized by gargling with water and mouth rinsing after pMDI use, or using a spacer device to facilitate less upper airway deposition.

5.2.2 **MDIs plus spacer**

A spacer device attached to a pMDI helps avoid problems in coordinating the timing of inhaler actuation and inhalation (Figure 5.3). It also overcomes the "cold freon" effect whereby the cold blast of propellant reaching the oropharynx results in cessation of inhalation or inhalation through the nose. If used correctly, a pMDI with spacer is at least as effective for delivery of inhaled drugs as any other device. Different manufacturers make different sizes of spacers and inhalers, although the following principles of use can be applied to most types:

- Ensure the inhaler fits snugly into the end of the spacer device
- Breathe out fully
- Put your lips around the mouthpiece

- Press the inhaler once
- Breath inwards fully and deeply
- Hold your breath for up to 10 seconds or as long as you find comfortable (alternatively take 5 normal breaths in and out)
- Repeat these steps if a second puff is required
- Wipe the mouthpiece clean.

Figure 5.3 A MDI with spacer

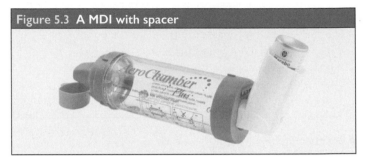

Aerosol drug particles delivered into a spacer may become lost to the chamber walls by electrostatic attraction between drug particles and chamber wall; this problem may be reduced by priming it 10–20 times or washing it. Spacers should generally be cleaned at least once a month with soapy water and allowed to drip dry. They should be replaced every 6–12 months, depending on the manufacturer's recommendations.

5.2.3 DPIs

DPIs used in asthma—examples include Accuhalers® and Turbohalers®—are breath activated. This means that the inspiratory flow rate generated by the patient de-aggregates the powder into smaller particles which are then dispersed within the lungs. The need for co-ordination is less than using a pMDI without a spacer and they are also less bulky and more portable. Different DPIs require different inspiratory flow rates (and higher flow rates than pMDIs) meaning that a more forceful inhalation is required to deposit the drug

Table 5.2 Approximate minimum inspiratory flow rates required to use different types of inhalers

Inhaler type	Minimum inspiratory flow rate (L/min)
Accuhaler®	30
Turbohaler®	30
Easi-Breathe® inhaler	20–30
Autohaler	20–30

within the lungs (Table 5.2). This in turn may influence which type of DPI is prescribed to a patient. Problems encountered with DPIs include failure to exhale to residual volume before use, exhaling into the mouthpiece after inhaling, inadequate or no breath hold, failure to hold the device upright and failure to inhale with sufficient force.

5.2.3.1 Accuhalers®

Accuhalers® (Figure 5.4) are manufactured to deliver SABAs, LABAs, ICSs, and LABAs and ICSs in combination to the lungs. To use an Accuhaler® correctly, patients should be instructed to:

- Open the device by pressing down on the thumb rest
- Click the lever down as far as possible
- Breathe out fully
- Put your lips around the mouthpiece and ensure a good seal
- Breathe inwards fully and deeply
- Hold your breath for up to 10 seconds or as long as you find comfortable
- Wipe the mouthpiece clean and close the device.

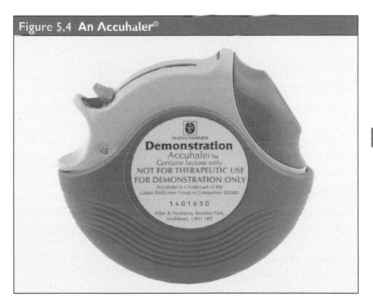

Figure 5.4 An Accuhaler®

5.2.3.2 Turbohalers®

Turbohalers® (Figure 5.5) are manufactured to deliver SABAs, LABAs, ICSs, and LABAs and ICSs in combination to the lungs. To use a Turbohaler® correctly, patients should be advised to take the following steps:

- Remove the outer cover
- Hold the inhaler upright
- Turn the base fully to the right and then back again until a click is heard
- Breathe out fully
- Put your lips around the mouthpiece and breathe inwards fully and deeply
- Hold your breath for up to 10 seconds or as long as you find comfortable
- Repeat these steps if a second puff is required
- Wipe the mouthpiece clean and replace the outer cover.

Figure 5.5 A Turbohaler®

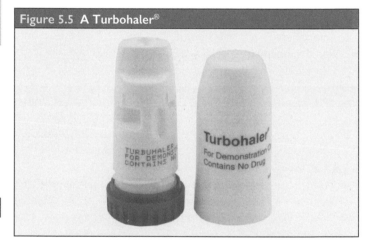

5.2.4 **Breath activated pMDIs**

These types of inhalers were developed in an attempt to overcome some of the problems associated with pMDIs. When a patient inhales through the trigger device, a mechanism automatically "fires" the breath activated MDI with the subsequent release of drug. This means that inhalation and actuation coincide with one another.

5.2.4.1 Easi-Breathe® inhalers

Easi-Breathe® inhalers (Figure 5.6) are manufactured to deliver SABAs and ICSs to the lungs. To use an Easi-Breathe® inhaler correctly, patients should be advised to take the following steps:

- Shake the inhaler
- Open the cap covering the mouthpiece

- Breathe out fully
- Put your lips around the mouthpiece and ensure a good seal (taking care not to block the air holes)
- Breathe inwards fully and deeply
- Hold your breath for up to 10 seconds or as long as you find comfortable
- Repeat these steps if a second puff is required
- Wipe the mouth piece clean and put the cap back over the mouthpiece.

Figure 5.6 An Easi-Breathe® inhaler

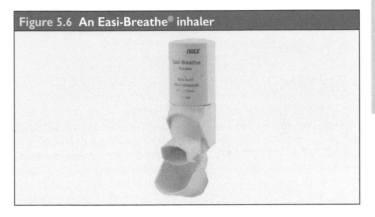

5.2.4.2 Autohalers

Autohalers (Figure 5.7) can deliver SABAs and ICSs to the lungs. To use an Autohaler correctly, patients should be advised to take the following steps:

- Shake the inhaler
- Open the cap covering the mouthpiece
- Breathe out fully
- Put your lips around the mouthpiece and ensure a good seal (taking care not to block the air holes)
- Breathe inwards fully and deeply
- Hold your breath for up to 10 seconds or as long as you find comfortable
- Repeat these steps if a second puff is required
- Wipe the mouthpiece clean and replace the cap.

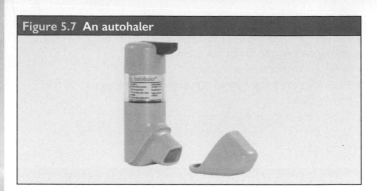

Figure 5.7 An autohaler

5.2.5 **Nebulizers**

Nebulizers, driven by compressed air or oxygen, create a mist of drug particle which is inhaled by the patient via a face mask or mouthpiece. They tend to be used during an acute episode of asthma, in either the primary or secondary care setting. Some patients with more severe asthma use a nebulizer on a domiciliary basis although the evidence behind this approach is lacking. Using a nebulizer is as effective as using a pMDI plus spacer correctly during an acute exacerbation. Despite delivering far higher doses than inhalers, nebulizers tend to be inefficient as most of the aerosol mist is lost to the atmosphere. Using a nebulizer can take as long as 10–20 minutes, while using an inhaler takes only a fraction of this time.

Further reading

British Thoracic Society/Scottish Intercollegiate Guideline Network. (2008) British guideline on the management of asthma. *Thorax* **63** (IV): i1–i121.

Broeders MEAC, Sanchis J, Levy ML, Crompton GK, Dekhuijzen PNR on behalf of the ADMIT Working Group (2009) The ADMIT series—Issues in Inhalation Therapy. 2) Improving technique and clinical effectiveness. *Prim Care Respir J* **18**: 76–82.

Lavorini F, Levy ML, Dekhuijzen PN, Crompton GK; ADMIT Working Group (2009) Inhaler choice and inhalation technique: key factors for asthma control. *Prim Care Respir J.* **18**: 241–2.

Chapter 6

Acute exacerbations

John F.W. Baker and Graeme P. Currie

Key points

- A variety of behavioural and psychological factors are associated with an increased risk of dying from an episode of acute asthma
- The main pharmacological adjuncts in the management of acute asthma consist of inhaled β_2-agonists, oral corticosteroids and oxygen in hypoxic patients
- Inhaled ipratropium, and intravenous magnesium sulphate (unlicensed indication) and aminophylline can be considered if a patient fails to adequately respond to initial treatment
- A high (or rise in) pCO_2 or low (or fall in) pH are ominous features; their presence should usually prompt discussion with intensive care.

6.1 Epidemiology

There has been an overall decrease in the number of hospital visits by patients with asthma in the past 20 years. However, this is mostly in the paediatric population, with rates of accident and emergency attendances and admission to hospital remaining much the same in adults. In 2009 there were over 61,000 admissions to hospital in England due to an acute exacerbation of asthma. These admissions alone cost the NHS around £45 million, although this figure fails to include prescription costs and lost productivity due to days off work. There has been a gradual decline in the number of deaths from acute asthma since the late 1980s, although this trend appears to be slowing. Around 1,400 individuals die each year of acute asthma in the UK, with more asthma deaths in younger populations in summer months, and a greater number of older individuals dying in winter.

The mean age of patients who required admission to hospital due to acute asthma in England in 2009 was 35. In the same year, over 15,000 of admissions in England were for patients over the age of 60.

Approximately half of these included patients over 75 years of age. Furthermore, over two-thirds of the deaths that occur as a result of asthma are in adults over 65 years of age.

6.2 **Aetiology**

Exacerbations of asthma can be caused by a variety of stimuli such as viral and bacterial infections, allergens, pollutants, some drugs and occupational exposures (Table 6.1); many however are due to poor or erratic concordance with anti-inflammatory treatment. Following all types of exposure, the end result is inflammatory cell influx and activation, exaggerated airway hyperresponsiveness, smooth muscle contraction and airflow obstruction, all of which leads to typical symptoms.

Table 6.1 Causes of exacerbations of asthma

Stimulus causing an exacerbation	Examples
Virus	Rhinovirus Respiratory syncytial virus Influenza Human metapneumovirus
Bacteria	*Mycoplasma pneumoniae* *Chlamydia pneumoniae* *Streptococcus pneumonia*
Allergens	Pollen Cat Dog House dust mite
Environmental pollutants	Cigarette smoke (active or passive) Sulphur dioxide Nitrogen dioxide Diesel fumes Ozone Particulate matter
Drugs	Aspirin NSAIDs β-blockers (including eye drops)
Occupational exposures	See Chapter 7

Many factors have been associated with an increased risk of having a fatal or near fatal episode of asthma (Box 6.1). It is therefore important that these factors are identified and recognized as a risk factor for mortality in those that present with an exacerbation. The appropriate management (where possible) of risk factors is desirable in reducing dependence on healthcare services and requirement for hospital admission.

Box 6.1 Medical and psychosocial features associated with a fatal or near fatal episode of asthma

Alcohol or drug abuse
Psychiatric illness
Denial
Non-concordance with prescribed medication
Learning difficulties
Frequent home visits
Fewer GP contacts
Inadequate follow-up
Increased use of reliever therapy
Inadequate use of oral or ICSs
Income and employment difficulties
Previous hospital self-discharge
Social isolation
Brittle asthma
Previous admission to intensive care for asthma

6.3 **Pathogenesis**

A variety of inflammatory cells, cytokines and mediators take part in a complex sequence of events to produce the vasodilatation, increased mucus secretion, oedema and bronchoconstriction that lead to features of an acute exacerbation of asthma. The complexity of the reaction is increased by the fact that many cytokines not only promote cellular activity but also have a direct effect on bronchial walls and vasculature. Post-mortem studies have shown that the cause of death in asthma is asphyxiation due to small airway obstruction. In such cases, a thickened and oedematous basement membrane becomes infiltrated with a variety of cell types, which produce a large amount of mucus and fibrin which is shed into the airway.

6.4 **Clinical features**

Patients tend to have limited perception of the severity of their asthma, which may in turn cause delay in seeking medical advice and result in clinicians underestimating the severity of an exacerbation.

Usual symptoms of an exacerbation are increased breathlessness, reduced exercise tolerance, cough (occasionally productive of yellow sputum), chest tightness, wheeze and increased β_2-agonist use. Some patients will have kept a record of PEF and will therefore be able to provide objective evidence of deteriorating asthma control. Indeed, all patients should be encouraged to do so in order to help recognize when their asthma is becoming less well controlled.

Clinical assessment is used not only to confirm the presence of an exacerbation but to assess severity, which in turn guides appropriate management (Table 6.2). The most commonly used parameters include:

- General observations such as central cyanosis, sweating, confusion, and coma
- PEF
- Ability to talk in sentences
- Respiratory rate
- Heart rate
- Blood pressure
- Accessory muscle use
- Chest signs
- Oxygen saturation.

Table 6.2 Clinical features of moderate, severe and life-threatening exacerbations of asthma

Feature	Moderate	Severe	Life-threatening
General	Breathless but able to complete whole sentences	Sitting forward, anxious, using accessory muscles, unable to complete sentences	Exhausted, confused, unable to speak, cyanosed, comatose, poor respiratory effort
PEF	>50–75% of best	33–50% of best	<33% of best or predicted
Respiratory rate	<25/min	≥25/min	Poor effort, low respiratory rate
Oxygen saturation	Usually >92%	Usually >92%	<92%
Pulse	<110/min	≥110/min	Bradycardia, arrhythmias
Chest signs	Expiratory wheeze	Expiratory wheeze	Silent chest

The use of pulsus paradoxus has been abandoned as it is both awkward to perform and adds little to assessment or subsequent management.

6.5 Investigations

Arterial blood gases should be performed if oxygen saturation is <92% (whether breathing room air or oxygen) or if there is evidence of a severe or life-threatening exacerbation. Repeat measurements may be required if the initial sample indicates a SpO_2 <92%, a PaO_2 <8 kPa, or if the $PaCO_2$ is normal or raised. In the majority of exacerbations requiring hospital admission, patients will have features of type 1 respiratory failure (Table 6.3). With clinical features of severe or life-threatening asthma, the presence of a high (or increasing) pCO_2 level and/or low (or decreasing) pH (type 2 respiratory failure) is an ominous feature and highlights the need for close monitoring and consideration of invasive ventilatory support. Moreover, a normal pCO_2 level provides little reassurance as the increased respiratory rate during an exacerbation should result in a reduction in pCO_2. In other words, if the pCO_2 level is within the normal range during an exacerbation of asthma, it may be an early indicator that the patient is becoming tired.

Table 6.3 Arterial blood gas features of type 1 and type 2 respiratory failure		
	Type 1 respiratory failure	**Type 2 respiratory failure**
pO_2	↓	↓
pCO_2	↔ or ↓	↑
HCO_3	↔	↑ or ↔
pH	↔ or ↑	↔ or ↓

Figure 6.1 Chest radiograph showing a right-sided pneumothorax in a patient admitted with a concomitant exacerbation of asthma

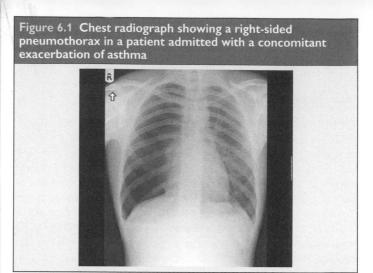

Figure 6.2 Chest radiograph showing a chest drain inserted into the right pleural cavity of the patient in Figure 6.1

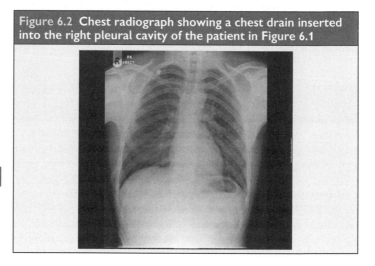

A chest radiograph is not required in all patients presenting with features of acute asthma. It should however usually be performed in patients with severe or life-threatening exacerbations, where consolidation or pneumothorax is suspected (Figures 6.1 and 6.2), when invasive ventilation is required or when the response to treatment is sub-optimal.

6.6 **Admission to hospital**

Up to 20% of all individuals presenting at an accident and emergency department are admitted to hospital. Those in the community or in the accident and emergency department who have a PEF >75% of personal best or predicted (before or 1 hour after treatment), may be allowed home so long as treatment for the exacerbation has been provided and advice given to seek further help in the event of a deterioration. However, other individuals with PEF >75% predicted may need to be admitted to hospital when there are concerns regarding compliance, social isolation, pregnancy, previous life-threatening episodes or persistent symptoms.

6.7 **Management**

The pivotal components of the management of acute asthma consist of inhaled bronchodilators, systemic corticosteroids and the administration of oxygen if hypoxic (Figure 6.3). The severity of the exacerbation will determine where treatment takes place (in primary care, accident and emergency departments, specialized respiratory wards or high dependency/intensive care units).

6.7.1 **Oxygen**
Many patients who present with acute severe asthma are hypoxaemic. Oxygen should be given to patients who have an exacerbation of asthma to maintain oxygen saturation ≥92% (preferably between 94–98%) with levels continuously monitored using a pulse oximeter.

Unlike COPD, there is less danger of high flow oxygen causing loss of hypoxic drive and subsequent CO_2 retention. However, there is concern that injudicious administration of high flow oxygen may mask a clinical deterioration despite maintenance of an oxygen saturation of 100%; in such individuals, a fall in oxygen saturation may herald a late and ominous feature of respiratory function.

6.7.2 **Inhaled bronchodilators**
Inhaled β_2-agonists underpin the management of all individuals with an exacerbation of asthma. Terbutaline and salbutamol are two available options although there is no evidence for greater efficacy between either β_2-agonist. Although a nebulizer does not confer any additional advantage in drug delivery over hand-held devices with a spacer, they are independent of patient effort and are more convenient in the busy ward or accident and emergency setting; 400 micrograms of salbutamol via a spacer device is equivalent to 2.5 mg of salbutamol delivered via a nebulizer. Salbutamol should

Figure 6.3 Algorithm showing the main steps involved in managing acute severe asthma in hospital

Immediate treatment

- Oxygen 40–60%
- Salbutamol 5mg or terbutaline 10 mg via an oxygen-driven nebulizer
- Ipratropium bromide 0.5 mg via an oxygen-driven nebulizer
- Oral prednisolone 40–50 mg or IV hydrocortisone 100 mg
- Chest X ray if pneumothorax or consolidation are suspected or patient requires mechanical ventilation

IF LIFE THREATENING FEAUTURES ARE PRESENT:

- Discuss with senior clinician
- IV magnesium sulphate (unlicensed indication) 1.2–2 g infusion over 20 minutes
- Nebulized salbutamol 5mg up to every 15–30 minutes

Subsequent Management

IF PATIENT IS IMPROVING CONTINUE:

- 40–60% oxygen
- Oral Prednisolone 40–50 mg daily or IV hydrocortisone 100 mg 6 hourly
- Nebulized β_2 agonist and ipratropium 4–6 hourly

IF PATIENT NOT IMPROVING AFTER 15–30 MINUTES:

- Continue oxygen and steroids
- Nebulized salbumatol 5 mg up to every 15–30 minutes
- Continue ipratropium 0.5 mg 4–6 hourly until patient is improving

IF PATIENT IS STILL NOT IMPROVING:

- Discuss patient with senior clinician
- IV magnesium sulphate (unlicensed indication) 1.2–2 g over 20 minutes (unless already given)
- Consider IV β_2 agonist/IV aminophylline/mechanical ventilation

Monitoring

- PEF 15–30 minutes after starting treatment
- Oximetry: maintain SpO_2 > 92%
- Repeat blood gas measurements within 2 hours of starting treatment if:
    - initial PaO_2 < 8 kPa (60 mmHg) unless subsequent SpO_2 > 92%
    - $PaCO_2$ normal or raised
    - patient deteriorates
- Chart PEF before and after giving β_2 agonists and at least 4 times daily throughout hospital stay

TRANSFER TO ICU ACCOMPANIED BY A DOCTOR PREPARED TO INTUBATE IF:

- Deteriorating PEF, worsening or persisting hypoxia, or hypercapnea
- Exhaustion, feeble respirations, confusion or drowsiness
- Coma or respiratory arrest

usually be given in repeated intervals of around 20 minutes depending on clinical response. In individuals with life-threatening asthma, continuous administration of nebulized salbutamol should be given at a dose of 5–10 mg/h. Where possible, nebulized β_2-agonists should be given through an oxygen-driven nebulizer due to the potential for oxygen desaturation in these patients. However, a lack of supplemental oxygen should not prevent the use of these medications when their use is indicated. Intravenous β_2-agonists may occasionally be used when effective nebulized treatment is not possible such as in ventilated patients or those in extremis.

Ipratropium has been shown to confer additive bronchodilator effects to those achieved by inhaled β_2-agonists alone. Nebulized ipratropium (500 micrograms) should therefore be considered in patients who fail to respond to inhaled salbutamol and should be repeated after a minimum of 60 minutes; subsequent treatment should be given every 4–6 hours.

6.7.3 Corticosteroids

Systemic corticosteroids are a fundamental component in the management of asthma exacerbations of any severity. They reduce mortality, relapse rate, and number of admissions as well as the requirement for β_2-agonists. Prednisolone 40–50 mg should be given orally for all patients at presentation and daily for at least 5 days, although 100 mg of intravenous hydrocortisone may be necessary if the patient is too breathless, unable to swallow or vomiting. Hydrocortisone has a shorter half-life than prednisolone and consequently more frequent doses will be required if this preparation is used. Oral prednisolone is well absorbed via the enteral route and its onset of action is the same as intravenous hydrocortisone; studies have generally shown that intravenous treatment confers little advantage over oral formulations.

Some data have suggested that high dose ICSs may be as effective as oral corticosteroids during acute exacerbations, although further trials are required to fully determine whether this should become part of standard treatment. Patients who already use, or who are started on ICSs, should continue these medications throughout their acute illness in order to maintain their chronic asthma management plan.

6.7.4 Magnesium

Magnesium causes relaxation of bronchial smooth muscle and subsequent bronchodilatation. It is now recommended in patients who fail to improve despite inhaled bronchodilators and systemic corticosteroids, especially those with acute severe asthma. However, a Cochrane meta-analysis of intravenous magnesium sulphate in acute asthma failed to demonstrate a beneficial effect in terms of improved lung function or reduced hospital admission rates, although some benefit was observed in those with a more severe exacerbation. In individuals presenting with a severe exacerbation, magnesium sulphate (unlicensed indication) should be given as a single dose of 1.2–2 g in 50–100 ml of 0.9% NaCl over 20 minutes; serum magnesium levels do not require to be measured before or after administration.

A solitary dose of IV magnesium sulphate is safe and may improve lung function in patients with acute severe asthma. However, the safety and efficacy of repeated doses has not yet been fully assessed. Repeated doses pose potential for hypermagnaesaemia and subsequent muscle weakness and respiratory failure.

6.7.5 **Aminophylline**

Aminophylline is a methyl xanthine and confers weak anti-inflammatory and bronchodilatory effects in asthma. Intravenous aminophylline is unlikely to lead to any significant additional benefits in comparison to standard care with inhaled bronchodilator therapy and corticosteroids. In a Cochrane meta-analysis evaluating the use of intravenous aminophylline in acute asthma, active treatment failed to confer any beneficial effects although it did result in a significant increase in vomiting, palpitations and arrythmias. Despite this, guidelines suggest that it may be used in individuals with severe and life-threatening disease who respond poorly to conventional treatment.

In patients not using an oral theophylline preparation, a loading dose of 5 mg/kg over at least 20 minutes should be given with cardiac monitoring with subsequent maintenance infusion of 500 micrograms/kg/h. In patients already using a theophylline preparation, the loading dose should be omitted and a plasma level should ideally be obtained prior to commencement of a maintenance infusion of 500 micrograms/kg/h. Plasma theophylline levels should be measured daily and the infusion rate altered to maintain a concentration between 10 and 20 mg/L (55–110 µmol/L). A variety of factors (Box 6.2) are associated with altering the plasma theophylline concentration.

6.7.6 **Antibiotics**

Most studies have demonstrated no significant benefit over standard care when antibiotics are added into the routine treatment algorithm. Antibiotics should only be used when there is objective evidence of bacterial infection such as chest radiograph consolidation, systemic features of sepsis or positive microbiological culture.

6.7.7 **LTRAs**

Leukotrienes can be found in the airway and urine following both spontaneous exacerbations of asthma and acute exposure to bronchoconstrictor stimuli in the laboratory. This in turn indicates that these inflammatory mediators may have a role in the pathogenesis of acute episodes of bronchoconstriction. Although LTRAs are not currently advocated in the management of acute asthma, there are

> **Box 6.2 Drugs and patient characteristics which alter plasma theophylline concentration**
>
> - Causes of increased plasma theophylline levels (i.e. reduced plasma clearance)
>   - Heart failure
>   - Liver cirrhosis
>   - Advanced age
>   - Ciprofloxacin
>   - Erythromycin
>   - Clarithromycin
>   - Verapamil
> - Causes of reduced plasma theophylline levels (i.e. increased plasma clearance)
>   - Cigarette smokers
>   - Chronic alcoholism
>   - Rifampicin
>   - Phenytoin
>   - Carbamazepine
>   - Lithium

data to suggest that they might be of some potential benefit. Indeed, some preliminary studies have demonstrated that LTRAs do confer some benefit when given at the time of an acute exacerbation, although further large-scale studies are required to confirm these observations.

6.7.8 **Non-invasive ventilation**

Non-invasive ventilation (NIV) is useful in patients with exacerbations of COPD who have decompensated hypercapnic respiratory failure. Few data are available to support its use in respiratory failure due to asthma and, as a consequence, intubation and mechanical ventilation remains the 'gold standard' approach. However, NIV may be considered in the intensive care or an appropriate clinical setting under specialized supervision, providing a low threshold exists towards switching to more conventional ventilation.

6.7.9 **Invasive ventilatory support**

Patients need to be considered for referral to the intensive care unit for consideration of invasive ventilation when they fail to respond to aggressive therapy. Typical clinical features that merit transfer include exhaustion with poor respiratory effort, respiratory arrest, confusion, drowsiness, deteriorating PEF, persisting hypoxia, hypercapnia or falling pH. Ideally the intensive care unit should be made aware of an individual with life-threatening features beforehand to allow a more smooth transition of care. Patients who have had a previous admission to the intensive care unit as a consequence of a life-threatening asthma exacerbation should be closely monitored due to the risks of a recurrent episode requiring this additional level of support.

6.7.10 **Subsequent management**

Oxygen should be continued to maintain saturation >92% (and preferably 94–98%). Oral prednisolone should usually be given for at least for 5 days (frequently 7 days); a tapering dose is not usually required. Inhaled (usually nebulized) salbutamol should be given 4–6 hourly as well as on an 'as required' basis. Individuals should remain on their usual maintenance inhalers throughout the treatment period. PEF measurements should be recorded up to four times daily to identify improvement objectively. Measurements should be taken before and after nebulized or inhaled therapy in order to assess response to treatment. Intravenous fluids should be given in dehydrated patients or to correct electrolyte imbalance. Consideration should be given to thromboprophylaxis with low molecular weight heparin in immobile patients and those at high risk of venous thromboembolism.

6.8 **Discharge planning**

Suitability for discharge depends on an improvement in clinical condition and varies between patients. Ideally, individuals should:

- Have a PEF >75% predicted
- Have a PEF diurnal variability <25%
- Have regular nebulized bronchodilators discontinued 24 hours prior to anticipated discharge
- Be requiring reducing amounts of inhaled β_2-agonists
- Be using maintenance inhalers
- Be receiving oral corticosteroids
- Have been reviewed by an asthma nurse and provided with a written action plan
- Be advised to attend their general practitioner or practice nurse within 2 days of discharge and be reviewed at a respiratory clinic within 4 weeks.

A diurnal variability of >25% or a PEF <75% are associated with an increased relapse rate and an increased rate of readmission and consequently are important markers of acute episode resolution.

6.9 **Prevention**

Avoiding exacerbations is centred around the use of optimal preventer therapy and the provision of comprehensive asthma education programmes comprising general information, self-monitoring of disease activity, regular medical or nursing reviews, and an individualized, written asthma action plan. These have been discussed in Chapter 3.

Further reading

Aldington S, Beasley R (2007) Asthma exacerbations: assessment and management of severe asthma in adults in hospital. *Thorax* **62**: 447–58.

British Thoracic Society/Scottish Intercollegiate Guideline Network. (2008) British guideline on the management of asthma. *Thorax* **63** (Suppl IV): i1–i121.

O'Driscoll BR, Howard LS, Davison AG (2008) BTS guideline for emergency oxygen use in adult patients. *Thorax* **63**: vi1–vi68.

Parameswaran K, Belda J, Rowe BH (2000) Addition of intravenous aminophylline to beta2-agonists in adults with acute asthma. *Cochrane Database of Systematic Reviews* 2000, Issue 4. Art. No.: CD002742. DOI: 10.1002/14651858.CD002742.

Ramsay CF, Pearson D, Mildenhall S, Wilson AM (2011) Oral montelukast in acute asthma exacerbations. a randomised, double-blind, placebo-controlled trial. *Thorax* **66**: 7–11.

Rowe BH, Bretzlaff J, Bourdon C, Bota G, Blitz S, Camargo CA (2000) Magnesium sulfate for treating exacerbations of acute asthma in the emergency department. *Cochrane Database of Systematic Reviews* 2000, Issue 1. Art. No.: CD001490. DOI: 10.1002/14651858.CD001490.

Chapter 7

Occupational asthma

Edward W. Paterson and Graeme P. Currie

Key points

- Occupational asthma causes up to 15% of new asthma occurring in adulthood
- The two main types of occupational asthma are classical occupational asthma (due to sensitization to a workplace exposure) and reactive airways dysfunction syndrome (RADS) (due to a single large exposure to an agent)
- Two-hourly PEF measurements provide a good way of confirming occupational asthma. Specific bronchial challenge is the 'gold standard' of determining a causal relationship but this is not routinely available
- In addition to standard pharmacological treatment, management includes avoidance of the causal agent, changes in work practice and provision of personal protective equipment. If these are ineffective or impossible, redeployment either within the same workplace or elsewhere may be necessary.

7.1 **Overview**

Occupational asthma is caused by exposure to agents in the workplace and is more common than usually appreciated. It accounts for 10–15% of new cases of asthma arising in those of working age. The two main types are classical sensitizing occupational asthma and RADS, which is due to a single large exposure to a chemical (such as a 'spill' at work). Both types need to be differentiated from asthma aggravated by work, which is observed in those with pre-existing asthma.

7.2 **Classical occupational asthma**

Patients with classical occupational asthma report symptoms with a work-related pattern; improvements are observed when away from work during weekends or holidays, although in some individuals such a clear association may not be immediately obvious. Clinicians should maintain a high level of suspicion that there could be an occupational cause to asthma when encountering any newly diagnosed adult. In individuals who work in a relatively high risk occupation, such as bakers and paint sprayers, the diagnosis should be positively sought. The key question when considering a diagnosis of occupational asthma is: are symptoms better at the weekends or holidays when away from work?

7.2.1 **Causes of occupational asthma**

Classical occupational asthma is caused by a sensitizing reaction in the airways to a specific 'asthmagen'. Occupational asthmagens (agents encountered at the workplace that cause occupational asthma) can be classified by molecular weight. Low molecular weight (<5000 Daltons) asthmagens largely consist of chemicals such as isocyanates, aldehydes, metals and drugs. High molecular weight (≥5000 Daltons) asthmagens are mostly proteins. Common examples of these include flour and grain dust, animal proteins (such as those found in rat urine), latex and enzymes used in baking or biological washing powders. There are currently over 400 recognized occupational asthmagens; some of the most commonly implicated agents and associated occupations are shown in Table 7.1.

Table 7.1 The most common agents known to cause classical occupational asthma in the UK and the most common occupations involved

Agent	Occupation
Isocyanates	Paint sprayers
Flour and grain	Bakers
Cutting oils and coolants	Engineering
Paints	Wide range of industries
Chrome compounds	Electroplaters, welders
Wood dust	Timber workers
Laboratory animal proteins	Laboratory workers
Acrylics and acrylates	Building industry, chemical processes
Solder, colophony	Plumbers, engineering workers
Enzymes, amylase	Washing powder manufacture, baking

7.2.2 **Pathogenesis**

Low molecular weight asthmagens do not directly result in the production of antibodies. They work by acting as haptens, which bind onto human proteins and are usually highly reactive compounds. There are certain molecular 'structure alerts' that are much more likely to do this. Typical examples include the isocyanate moiety (–N=C=O), primary and secondary amines, dicarboxylic acid anhydrides and dialdehydes. These agents may be implicated in paint sprayers, solderers and cleaners, epoxy resin workers and hospital staff, respectively.

High molecular weight agent asthmagens usually exert their effects through an immunoglobulin (Ig) E response. The majority tend to be proteins or glycoproteins of animal or vegetable origin. In some situations the agent contains intrinsic enzymatic activity such as alcalase in occupational asthma due to detergents. As a result of their own enzymatic activity, they may potentiate allergenicity of the molecule itself by disrupting tight junctions between cells.

7.2.3 **Clinical features**

Symptoms of occupational asthma are similar to those of typical asthma. Patients commonly report wheeze, chest tightness, breathlessness and cough when exposed to the responsible asthmagen. An accurate occupational history is fundamental and should include details of all previous and current jobs, which allows assessment of exposure to known asthmagens. Knowledge of each job since leaving school enables both the identification of unsuspected exposures and determines the latent period prior to the development of symptoms, as most cases occur within 2 years of first exposure to the relevant agent. Symptoms being better away from work (either at the weekend or for longer periods away such as on holiday) provide the first clue that the patient may have occupational asthma. In some cases symptoms are worse in the evening after exposure, and a work-related pattern can therefore be easily missed. This is due to the late phase immunological reaction observed with some exposures.

Knowledge that other individuals at the same workplace have work-related symptoms or overt occupational asthma is also helpful, although this is usually not apparent at first presentation. A possible diagnosis of occupational asthma should be investigated as soon as the possibility has arisen, as removal from the source is the most effective treatment and persistent exposure may result in irreversible symptoms.

7.2.4 **Diagnosis**

Diagnosing occupational asthma depends on demonstrating characteristic patterns of lung function—usually PEF—variation with exposure (Figure 7.1). Occasionally, serial FEV_1 across a work shift where exposure occurs is used. PEF measurements are easy to arrange, simple to perform and are cheap; disadvantages include erratic compliance and discrepancies in the recording of accurate values.

To diagnose occupational asthma, the PEF should ideally be measured:

- Every 2 hours from wakening to sleeping
- Over 5 weeks during a period of unaltered asthma pharmacotherapy (with the exception of 'as required' use of SABAs which should be recorded)
- For at least 3 days during each work period
- With at least three series of consecutive work days and three periods away from the workplace
- Incorporating a 1-week period away from work

Evaluation of PEF recordings can be carried out using a computer programme (OASYS) that accurately interprets serial measurements and calculates variability in readings (Figure 7.1). However, analysis

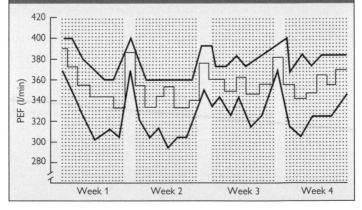

Figure 7.1 2 hourly **PEF** recordings in a textile worker; shaded areas represent days of exposure and clear areas time away from work. For each day, the maximum, minimum and mean **PEF** values are plotted. During exposure, the **PEF** fell and subsequently recovered when away from exposure. In the last week, although still at work, the individual was not exposed to material dust explaining why **PEF** recordings were relatively well maintained.

of data by an experienced clinician remains a prerequisite in overall assessment.

Where PEF monitoring is unreliable or cannot be performed, non-specific airway hyperresponsiveness can be measured using increasing concentrations of inhaled methacholine or histamine. A greater than 3.2-fold difference (in values when at work versus when away from work) in provocative concentration of methacholine causing a 20% fall in FEV_1 is regarded as being significant. However, not all individuals with occupational asthma demonstrate airway hyperresponsiveness to methacholine. When no longer exposed, airway hyperresponsiveness usually resolves over a 2–3-year period.

When doubt remains as to the true causal relationship between a suspected agent and asthma symptoms, a specific airway challenge to the suspected asthmagen may be undertaken. This is regarded as the gold standard in the diagnosis of occupational asthma but is not widely available.

7.2.5 Management

The occupational physician should identify responsible asthmagens and then remove the worker from exposure. In some cases this will depend upon reducing exposure to a level at which sensitization or the development of asthma is unlikely to occur. However, in only a very few cases is there sufficient evidence to support a clear threshold below which sensitization will not occur. The best approach is to remove the particular asthmagen completely and find a substitute material to work with. When this is impractical, for instance in baking where the agent cannot be replaced, changes in work practice might reduce exposure. As a last resort, personal protective equipment should be provided, for instance as in laboratory animal and pharmaceutical workers. If all these measures fail or are impossible, the worker may have to be relocated or move to a different job. Replacement of the relevant agent can be very effective in some workplaces, such as the observed fall in latex asthma in healthcare workers with the introduction of latex- and powder-free gloves. Rates of glutaraldehyde asthma were markedly reduced by the introduction of enclosed sterilizing units in endoscopy suites and theatres.

In the UK, Control of Substances Hazardous to Health (COSHH) regulations mean that employers are required to document all agents that workers are exposed to and any associated risk to health. Under the Reporting of Injuries, Diseases and Dangerous Occurrences Regulations (RIDDOR) employers are also requested to report cases of occupational asthma once confirmed.

The pharmacological treatment of occupational asthma is essentially the same as typical asthma. This includes the initial use of intermittent SABAs and then adding in regular ICSs with the consideration of LABAs in those with persistent symptoms.

7.2.6 **Prognosis**

If removed from exposure, the outlook is good for many individuals, but in some, the condition persists despite removal. In some exposures (notably isocyanates), accelerated loss of lung function can occur even after removal from the cause.

Occupational asthma is costly. The main financial burden is borne equally between the patient and state, with employers bearing very little. The exception to this is in specific instances where major changes to the workplace are required.

7.3 **RADS**

RADS occurs generally as a consequence of a large, single exposure to gas, vapour or fumes. However, more diffuse sources such as the dust from the destruction of the World Trade Centre has also resulted in this condition. The commonest recorded agent causing RADS is chlorine gas.

Individuals will not have had previous respiratory symptoms (although some accept the diagnosis in patients who have had prior symptoms) and atopy is usually absent. Symptoms typically develop within 24 hours of exposure and non-specific airway hyperresponsiveness must persist for at least 3 months. Patients with RADS complain of similar symptoms to those with typical asthma, although cough is frequently a dominant feature. In RADS, spirometry may be normal or obstructive but non-specific airway hyperresponsiveness to methacholine is the cardinal feature. A diagnosis of RADS is difficult to sustain without this.

The treatment of RADS is similar to that of other forms of asthma, although patients may be significantly less responsive to β_2-agonists and ICSs. The more long-term clinical outcome of RADS is poorly understood and individuals may demonstrate persistent airway hyperresponsiveness and have symptoms for many years following exposure.

7.4 **Work-aggravated asthma**

It is often difficult to distinguish true occupational asthma from pre-existing asthma which is aggravated by the work environment. For example, stimuli such as exercise, dust, cold air and tobacco smoke can induce or exacerbate symptoms in asthmatics who would not usually be exposed to such agents at home. This is often just as difficult a problem for the work occupational physician to deal with as classical occupational asthma. The aim is to reduce the relevant exposure in order to maintain the worker's health and work efficiency.

7.5 **Legal issues**

In many countries, classical occupational asthma is a compensatable disease for which the government provides a pension, but this may not apply to RADS. In some cases, workers need to consider civil law approaches in order to achieve redress. Work-aggravated asthma is not compensatable.

Further reading

Cowl CT (2011).Occupational asthma: review of assessment, treatment, and compensation. *Chest* **139**: 674–81.

Newman Taylor AJ, Nicholson PJ, eds (2004) *Guidelines for the Prevention, Identification and Management of Occupational Asthma: evidence review and recommendations*. British Occupational Health Research Foundation, London. http://www.occupationalasthma.com.

Rachiotis G, Savani R, Brant A, MacNeill SJ, Taylor AN, Cullinan P. (2007) Outcome of occupational asthma after cessation of exposure: a systematic review. *Thorax* **62**: 147–52.

Chapter 8

Asthma in special circumstances

Pratheega Mahendra, John F.W. Baker, and
Graeme P. Currie

Key points

- During pregnancy, the clinical control of asthma is
  said to improve in one-third, remain the same in
  one-third and deteriorate in one-third
- The general principles of asthma management are the
  same in pregnant as in non-pregnant women
- Drugs used in the management of acute and chronic
  asthma are generally safe for use in pregnancy
- During an acute exacerbation of asthma in pregnancy,
  hypoxia and hypotension should be aggressively
  managed; early obstetric and intensive care advice
  should be obtained where necessary
- Individuals with features of active asthma should
  avoid underwater diving
- Most patients with asthma can fly in commercial
  aircraft without risk of adverse event; some
  hypoxic patients with advanced disease may
  require supplemental in-flight oxygen.

8.1 **Pregnancy**

Asthma is one of the most common chronic conditions that affect
women during pregnancy (4–12% of pregnancies). When asthma is
poorly controlled, there are potentially serious consequences for
both the mother and the unborn child. Retrospective studies have
indicated that uncontrolled asthma can be associated with adverse
outcomes in pregnancy such as pre-term birth, low birth weight and
pre-eclampsia. The risk is 15–20% higher than in a non-asthmatic
woman. This increases further to 30–100% in more severe asthma.
It is often quoted that the clinical control of asthma improves in

about one-third of women during pregnancy, remains the same in one-third and deteriorates in one-third, although it is more likely to deteriorate in those with more severe disease. The reasons for this and the mechanisms involved remain to be elucidated.

A number of factors that are likely to influence the course of asthma during pregnancy are known. For example:

- The maternal immune system is altered during pregnancy, so that the foetus (genetically different) does not undergo immunological rejection
- The presence of a female foetus is associated with worsening of asthma control
- a perception commonly exists that medication during pregnancy harms the foetus (this may lead to reduced compliance with ICSs)
- poorly controlled or severe asthma is associated with greater frequency of exacerbations and poorer asthma control during pregnancy
- modified cell-mediated immunity during pregnancy may alter the maternal response to inflammation and susceptibility to infection
- cigarette smoking and obesity contribute to deteriorating asthma control during pregnancy.

8.1.1 **Diagnosis**

In the majority of cases this is straightforward due to an antecedent diagnosis of asthma. However, further testing may be indicated in patients who have not previously received a diagnosis or asthma, or in those that present atypically. The most common differential diagnosis in these patients is dyspnoea of pregnancy. Unlike asthma, this does not typically present with cough, chest tightness, airflow obstruction or wheeze. Other potential alternative diagnoses are the same as in non-pregnant patients: bronchitis, laryngeal dysfunction, hyperventilation, chronic cough and gastro-oesophageal reflux. Given the increased risk of thromboembolic disease in pregnancy and immediately post-partum, pulmonary embolism is also an important consideration.

Diagnostic criteria are the same for pregnant women as for anyone with asthma. It is worth noting that methacholine testing to identify bronchial hypersensitivity is contraindicated in pregnancy due to lack of data regarding its safety. Previously undiagnosed asthmatics should undergo blood testing for specific IgE antibodies to common household allergens. However, skin testing is generally not advocated as it may be associated with systemic reactions, endangering both maternal and fetal health.

As in any patient with asthma, spirometry is the gold standard for assessing pulmonary function. However, serial twice a day peak flow measurements may provide a straightforward and acceptable alternative. Standardised values for PEF and FEV_1 do not change significantly as a result of pregnancy and predicted and previous measurements can still be used in overall assessment. Measurement of fractioned exhaled nitric oxide (FE(NO)) could also be used since it is not influenced by pregnancy.

8.1.2 Clinical features

Clinicians should be aware that clinical features of asthma are similar in the pregnant and non-pregnant state. Ideally, pregnant women with asthma should be assessed every month. During a consultation, it is helpful to determine level of asthma control, through both subjective and objective means. Inadequate control may be indicated by the presence of daytime and nocturnal symptoms and increased frequency of reliever use. Some patients have a reduced perception of symptoms of significant airflow obstruction and in certain circumstances it is useful to monitor control by daily PEF recordings. A diurnal variation of greater than 20% is regarded as significant and suggests less well controlled asthma.

8.1.3 Acute asthma

Acute exacerbations of asthma are more likely to occur towards the end of the second or third trimester, although they are less common during labour. The diagnosis of acute asthma will more likely be made in a patient with known disease, although it can present for the first time during pregnancy. Recent prospective studies have shown that where exacerbations are managed appropriately, there is no excess risk of pregnancy complications, which in turn emphasizes the importance of rapid assessment and adequate treatment.

In pregnant women admitted to hospital for suspected acute asthma, the diagnosis rests heavily on history and examination findings. It is important to remember that breathlessness in a pregnant woman with a history of asthma is not always due to heightened airway inflammation and bronchoconstriction. The differential diagnosis includes:

- Pulmonary embolism
- Pneumothorax
- Pneumonia
- Hyperventilation (whether due to anxiety or physiological response to pregnancy)
- Amniotic fluid embolism
- Peripartum cardiomyopathy
- Pulmonary oedema.

In some cases a chest radiograph is indicated to rule out other potential diagnoses such as pneumothorax or pneumonia. The dose of radiation involved in a single chest radiograph is small and where the potential risk of missing other diagnoses outweighs any risks to the foetus, expectant mothers should not be declined this investigation.

8.1.4 **Management**

The aim of treatment of chronic asthma during pregnancy is to produce a situation where the patient has minimal or no symptoms and does not require regular use of β_2-agonists to relieve symptoms. General measures involved in overall management include patient education, smoking cessation advice, avoidance of trigger factors where possible and relaxation techniques. The guidelines for the use of asthma medication during pregnancy is largely unchanged from those for adults in general (Table 8.1).

Table 8.1 Managing asthma during pregnancy and lactation		
Severity	**PEFR (vs predicted)**	**Recommendation**
Mild/intermittent (<2 days/week)	≥80%	No daily medication needed.
Mild/persistent (>2 days/week, < daily)	≥80%	Low-dose ICS
Moderate (daily)	≥60%, <80%	EITHER • Low-dose ICS and LABA OR • Medium-dose ICS If needed • Medium-dose ICS and LABA
Severe (continual)	<60%	High-dose ICS AND • LABA AND, if needed, • Oral corticosteroids
		Theophylline/LTRA may be considered as second-line treatments in severe asthma

During an acute exacerbation, an important aim is to avoid hypoxic or hypotensive episodes in the expectant mother (which may potentially harm the foetus) with the use of high flow oxygen and intravenous fluids where necessary. Target oxygen saturations are 94–98%. It might also be necessary to place some patients in the left lateral position to reduce pressure on the inferior vena cava from a gravid uterus or preferably in a seated rather than supine position, since peak expiratory flow rates and FEV$_1$ are lower during pregnancy when supine. Exacerbations should generally be treated aggressively, and early contact made with the intensive care unit and obstetrician where necessary. Clinicians and expectant mothers alike should be aware that drugs used in the management of acute and chronic asthma are generally safe for use in pregnancy, and the risks of poorly controlled asthma far outweigh any potential risk arising from most treatments.

Continuous fetal monitoring is recommended in patients suffering with acute severe asthma during pregnancy, especially in the second and third trimesters. Current guidelines for the management of asthma during pregnancy suggest that there should be close liaison between the respiratory physician and the obstetrician for patients with poorly controlled disease.

8.1.5 **ICSs**

Extensive experience with and surveillance of ICSs during pregnancy have indicated their safety. ICSs are not generally absorbed into the body in any significant quantities, while the enzyme 11β-hydroxysteroid dehydrogenase in the placenta metabolizes a variety of corticosteroids, including betamethasone, beclometasone, dexamethasone and prednisolone. Fluticasone and budesonide are not metabolized by this enzyme, but studies have not shown any adverse effects on the foetus due to these drugs. Women with asthma using ICSs should therefore be encouraged to continue taking them throughout pregnancy. It is important to assess compliance, since studies show decreased inhaled steroid compliance in early pregnancy compared to pre pregnancy, possibly due to patients' concerns regarding drug safety.

8.1.6 **Oral corticosteroids**

Oral corticosteroids have been implicated in causing a slight increase in the rate of cleft palate in children born to mothers who received them in the first trimester. Palatal closure is completed by the 12th week of pregnancy so the potential risk would be limited to administration during the first trimester. However, it is difficult to tease out in studies whether it was the use of oral corticosteroids or the severity of asthma that caused the increased incidence of the abnormality. Moreover, in one study there were reasons other than asthma for taking corticosteroids and the duration of oral corticosteroid use was longer than is generally used for acute asthma. Whatever the cause of the association, the absolute increase in risk of cleft palate is small (0.1% to 0.3%). It is also possible that oral corticosteroid use in pregnancy can result in lower birth weight children. In general, it seems sensible to treat asthma exacerbations with short courses of prednisolone as for non-pregnant patients, as the risks of uncontrolled exacerbations are likely to be greater than any harm to the foetus.

8.1.7 β$_2$-agonists

Large studies have indicated that β$_2$-agonists are generally safe during pregnancy and breastfeeding. In one study, the use of SABAs during pregnancy seemed to have a beneficial effect by decreasing the risk of pregnancy induced hypertension. However, LABAs (salmeterol, formoterol) should only be used in combination with an ICS (i.e. not as monotherapy) where the latter alone has failed to control symptoms.

8.1.8 **LTRAs**

Animal data have indicated that LTRAs are not likely to be teratogenic, although data in human pregnancies have so far been limited to small studies. However, the available literature in humans suggests that these drugs do not confer adverse effects either on the foetus or the course of pregnancy. Also, emerging evidence particularly about montelukast is reassuring, therefore, if required, montelukast should be used in preference to other LTRAs. At present, the recommendation is that LTRAs should not be initiated during pregnancy, but may be continued if a patient has severe asthma not adequately controlled on ICSs and LABAs.

8.1.9 **Methylxanthines**

Theophylline and aminophylline are not contraindicated in pregnancy. Target theophylline plasma levels should be 8–12 mcg/ml rather than 10–15 mcg/ml since decreased binding to albumin results in increased proportion of free drug in the circulation. Clearance of theophylline appears to decrease during the 3rd trimester, therefore requiring decreased maintenance dose.

8.1.10 **Other drugs**

Inhaled ipratropium and intravenous magnesium sulphate (unlicensed indication) are safe in pregnancy.

8.1.11 **Managing asthma during labour**

The use of regular asthma medication should be continued throughout the obstetric period. Mothers receiving a dose of oral prednisolone greater than 7.5 mg per day during the 2 week period prior to labour should receive addition steroid cover during labour. The dose should be 100 mg of intravenous hydrocortisone 6–8 hourly during this period. This should continue for first 24 hours following delivery to prevent adrenal crisis.

In the event that anaesthesia is required for these patients during labour, regional blockade may be preferable to general anaesthesia. Oxygen consumption and minute ventilation have been shown to decrease following lumbar anaesthesia.

Care should be taken with the use of prostaglandins for cervical ripening, the management of induced or spontaneous abortions, or in postpartum haemorrhage. Prostaglandins E_1 and E_2 can be used safely, although close attention should be paid to respiratory status throughout. Prostaglandin $F_{2\alpha}$ should be avoided or used with extreme caution due to the significantly increased risk of bronchoconstriction that it carries.

8.1.12 Breastfeeding

Only small amounts of asthma medications in regular use have been found to enter into breast milk. Breast feeding should therefore be encouraged in all women, irrespective of their asthma severity.

8.2 Underwater diving

British Thoracic Society guidelines on respiratory aspects of fitness for diving indicate that patients with asthma should be advised *not* to dive if they have wheeze precipitated by exercise, cold or emotion. However, individuals with asthma may be permitted to dive—with or without regular anti-inflammatory treatment—if they have:

- No symptoms of active asthma
- Normal spirometry
- A negative exercise test (regarded as a less than 15% fall in FEV_1 following exercise).

The guidelines further suggest that they should also monitor their asthma with twice daily PEF recordings, and avoid diving if they have:

- Active asthma (defined as symptoms requiring relief medication in 48 hours preceding a dive)
- Reduced PEF (>10% fall from best values)
- Increased PEF variability (>20% diurnal variability).

8.3 Flying

Most individuals with asthma can safely fly and are not expected to experience any adverse effects from doing so. It is important that patients take reliever inhalers onto the flight with hand luggage, while nebulizers may be used at the discretion of the particular airline. Some patients with asthma who experience frequent exacerbations may find it useful to take a short course of prednisolone for use in an emergency when travelling abroad.

A small proportion of individuals with chronic asthma, especially elderly patients with advanced disease and a previous history of smoking, may be hypoxic while breathing room air (21% oxygen). Even in healthy subjects, the partial pressure of oxygen falls at altitude, which might compound any respiratory difficulties encountered with a hypoxaemic individual during a flight. Commercial aircraft are pressurized to a cabin pressure of 2,438 m (8,000 feet), at which the partial pressure in arterial blood falls to the equivalent of breathing approximately 15% oxygen at sea level. In patients who have an adequate partial oxygen pressure at sea level, oxygenation may fall below desirable levels when cabin altitude is simulated. This desaturation is exacerbated by minimal exercise.

In potentially hypoxic patients, the oxygen saturation on air using a pulse oximeter should be measured before flights are booked. This in turn will help determine whether in-flight oxygen is required or not (Table 8.2). All individuals who require in-flight oxygen should inform the relevant airline when booking and be aware that some airlines charge for this service. Moreover, any need for oxygen on the ground and while changing flights must also be considered.

Table 8.2 Advice regarding necessity (or otherwise) of in-flight oxygen in commercial aircraft

Oxygen saturation on air	Recommendation
>95%	Oxygen not required
92–95% (without risk factor*)	Oxygen not required
92–95% (with risk factor*)	Hypoxic challenge test[†]
<92%	In-flight oxygen required (2 or 4 L/min)
Already receiving long-term oxygen therapy	Increase flow rate

* Risk factor: FEV_1 <50% predicted, lung cancer, respiratory muscle weakness and other restrictive ventilatory disorders, within 6 weeks of hospital discharge.

[†] This involves subjects breathing 15% oxygen at sea level to mimic the environment with reduced inspiratory oxygen pressure to which they would be exposed during a typical commercial flight. Those with pO_2 >7.4 kPa post hypoxic challenge do not require in-flight oxygen, those with pO_2 <6.6 kPa require in-flight oxygen, and those with pO_2 6.6–7.4 kPa are considered borderline.

Further reading

British Thoracic Society recommendations (2002) Managing passengers with respiratory disease planning air travel. *Thorax* **57**: 289–304.

Blais L, Beauchesne MF, Rey E, Malo JL, Forget A. (2007) Use of inhaled corticosteroids during the first trimester of pregnancy and the risk of congenital malformations among women with asthma. *Thorax* **62**: 320–8.

Godden D, Currie GP, Denison D, *et al.* (2003) The British Thoracic Society guidelines on respiratory aspects of fitness for diving. *Thorax* **58**: 3–13.

Murphy VE, Clifton VL, Gibson PG. (2006) Asthma exacerbations during pregnancy: incidence and association with adverse pregnancy outcomes. *Thorax* **61**: 169–76.

Rey E, Boulet L (2007) Asthma in pregnancy. *Br Med J* **334**: 582–5.

Schatz M. Dombrowski MP (2009) Asthma in Pregnancy *NEJM* **360**; 18 (1862–9).

Chapter 9

Paediatric asthma: epidemiology and aetiology

Steve Turner

Key points

- Childhood asthma is a common condition in the UK and around the world
- Asthma is a complex condition and aetiology involves a series of interactions between genetic and environmental factors, often occurring in early life
- Early life exposures are associated with early onset symptoms which often persist
- Predicting asthma outcome is difficult, although coexisting allergy is the best predictor of symptoms persisting.

9.1 Introduction

The study of childhood asthma remains a challenge given the absence of definition and diagnostic test. Despite the lack of gold standard for diagnosis, researchers continue to describe trends in childhood asthma and the underlying mechanisms.

9.2 A historical backdrop

The word 'asthma' itself is a misnomer and is a Greek word describing a state of breathlessness or panting. Hippocrates used the word asthma interchangeably with orthopnoea and dyspnoea. Descriptions of cases consistent with asthma are found throughout Greek, Roman, Arabic and mediaeval European texts and it appears that asthma symptoms have been recognized for many thousands of years.

9.3 **Epidemiology**

The widely-reported asthma epidemic took place during the 1980s and 1990s; more recent surveys of populations in the UK indicate that the prevalence may be falling in the population. Asthma prevalence has been ascertained in Aberdeen school children beginning in 1964 when the lifetime prevalence was 4%. In the 2004 survey lifetime asthma prevalence was 28% and this had fallen to 22% in 2009. Worldwide, the prevalence of asthma varies between 1 and 30% and there is evidence of some countries having 'come through' the epidemic and others still experiencing increasing prevalence. Asthma symptoms are more common in boys compared to girls. This gender difference narrows as puberty approaches and they eventually reverse with women subsequently having a higher asthma prevalence compared to men. Asthma is more common in younger children and although symptoms apparently resolve in many, episodic wheeze recurs in adulthood in approximately 25%.

Asthma is associated with allergic conditions such as eczema, hay fever and food allergy but the relationship between asthma and allergy is not straightforward since most allergic individuals do not have asthma and approximately 20% of children with asthma are not allergic. There is a strong hereditary component to asthma: identical twins are more concordant for asthma compared to fraternal twins, and genetic factors are thought to explain approximately 50% of asthma causation. There is no single asthma gene; instead there are approximately ten genes each making a modest contribution towards asthma risk and these differ between populations. The remainder of asthma causation is explained by environmental factors and these appear to include exposure to tobacco smoke, diet (in particular maternal diet during pregnancy), exposure to 'dirt', *in utero* growth retardation, breast feeding, infection with respiratory viruses, day care, birth order and obesity, although this list is not exhaustive. Genetic predispositions in combination with environmental exposures occurring at certain critical times (often in the first two years of life) are implicated in asthma causation.

9.4 **Aetiology**

The reasons for the dramatic rise and apparent fall in childhood asthma prevalence are not well understood but genetic variation in the population cannot explain such a rapid surge in prevalence. The International Study of Asthma and Allergy in Children demonstrated highest prevalence of asthma in Western countries including UK, Australia, New Zealand and USA, suggesting an association between asthma and a 'Westernized lifestyle.' This was confirmed after the fall of the Iron curtain in the 1990s where there were rises in asthma prevalence among children in East Germany to values seen in Western German peers. What constitutes a 'Western lifestyle' remains to be defined. A number of related hypotheses have been proposed including the hygiene and dietary hypotheses. Children who have older siblings are at reduced risk for allergic conditions (although not asthma in most surveys) and this observation led to the hygiene hypothesis being proposed, i.e. exposure to infections contracted from older siblings during early life may protect against the development of allergy. The hygiene hypothesis has been mis-interpreted and linked to the concept that increased use of deter-gents and general cleanliness in modern homes may expose very young infants to an environment which favours the development of an 'allergic' immune system; there is limited evidence to support this variant of the hygiene hypothesis.

There is substantial literature to support the role of early respira-tory infection in the later development of asthma; in particular, the common cold virus is implicated. The dietary hypothesis proposes that an excess of dietary oxidant or lack of dietary antioxidants in maternal diet during pregnancy lead to increased asthma. There is some evidence to support this and the UK population's dietary anti-oxidant intake, for example vitamin E, fell during the asthma epidemic but intervention studies, where mothers are randomized to nutrient-augmented diet or not, are required to test this hypothesis.

The fetal origins hypothesis proposes that antenatal stresses result in fetal growth failure followed by physiological and/or metabolic changes which allow the fetus to survive to term but at the expense of increased risk for chronic illnesses in later life. Observation stud-ies where fetal ultrasound measurements are linked to asthma out-comes in childhood provide some evidence to support the early origins hypothesis, in addition to the large evidence base linking reduced birth weight to increased asthma risk. These hypotheses, and others implicating antenatal exposures to paracetamol and products of tobacco smoke, place exposures in early life as crucial to asthma causation and this is consistent with the observation that many children with asthma are initially symptomatic in preschool years. Other factors which may also be related to asthma causation include a sedentary lifestyle, obesity, and indoor and outdoor air quality. In adults, occupational exposures are important. There are some children in whom symptoms begin later in life and different factors have been implicated in children with different patterns of symptoms or 'phenotypes'.

Perhaps the greatest insight into asthma aetiology comes from intervention studies where infants usually at high risk for develop-ing asthma have their environment modified. These studies have not always provided what was expected. Researchers in the Isle of

Wight modified infants' diets and reduced house dust mite exposure and their intervention was associated with reduced asthma. In contrast, researchers in Manchester found that reduced house dust mite exposure was associated with less obstructed lung function but increased allergy to house dust mite. A third group in Belarus found that prolonged breast feeding was associated with increased allergy but not reduced asthma. These studies confirm that asthma is complex and influenced by exposures in early life. These studies also give insight into the inconsistent relationship between asthma and allergy.

9.5 **When do the physiological and pathological changes associated with asthma begin?**

Childhood asthma is associated with airflow obstruction on spirometry, bronchial hyper-reactivity and airway inflammation and thickening of the epithelial basement membrane on biopsy. What has been demonstrated is that airflow obstruction is present shortly after birth in infants who later go on to develop asthma and bronchial hyper-reactivity develops during infancy before the onset of symptoms. In contrast, the epithelial basement membrane thickening is not present in infants with persistent wheeze but is established in three year olds with asthma-like symptoms. These findings suggest that some features of asthma are present at birth but others develop during the first few years of life. This paradigm is consistent with childhood asthma being caused by a series of 'hits' (i.e. gene environment interactions) during the early years of life.

9.6 **Natural history during childhood— phenotypes**

There are some children in whom early asthma symptoms resolve, others in whom symptoms persist and yet others with new onset asthma as they approach puberty. These different age-related patterns or 'phenotypes' give some insight into asthma causation but have little clinical relevance since individuals rarely fit neatly into one of the phenotypes; all have similar symptoms and respond to the same treatments. Children who grow out of early asthma symptoms are more likely to be male and have smoking mothers, whereas those with later onset symptoms are more likely to have hay fever and eczema. Children whose early onset wheeze persists are intermediate between early onset and late onset asthma, i.e. more likely to have mothers who smoked and to have hay fever and eczema. Children with asthma symptoms and negative skin prick tests are more likely to grow out of their symptoms. Together, these observations suggest that different combinations of factors may result in asthma persistence.

9.7 **Childhood asthma beyond childhood**

Follow up of children with asthma demonstrates that symptoms remit in many individuals, but approximately 25% who have apparently grown out of their asthma experience symptoms in adulthood. Many adults with clinical remission of childhood asthma symptoms continue to exhibit the physiological abnormalities found in symptomatic asthmatics. The more severe asthmatic children tend to have persistent symptoms, and factors such as reduced FEV_1 and atopy in childhood are associated with increased risk for persistence of symptoms.

Further reading

Asher MI, Montefort S, Björkstén B, Lai CKW, Strachan DP, Weiland SK, Williams H, and the ISAAC Phase Three Study Group (2006) Worldwide time trends in the prevalence of symptoms of asthma, allergic rhinoconjunctivitis, and eczema in childhood: ISAAC Phases One and Three repeat multicountry cross sectional surveys. *Lancet* **368**(9537): 733–43.

Eder W, Ege MJ, von Mutius E.(2006) The asthma epidemic. *N Engl J Med* **355**: 2226–35.

McLeish S, Turner SW (2008) Gene-environment interactions in asthma. *Arch Dis Child* **92**: 1032–5.

Phelan PD, Robertson CF, Olinsky A (2002) The Melbourne Asthma Study: 1964–1999 *J Allergy Clin Immunol* **109**: 189–94.

Chapter 10

Paediatric asthma: diagnosis

Steve Turner

Key points

- Viral induced wheeze is the most common differential diagnosis for wheeze in children
- It is important to clarify the true nature of 'wheeze' since rattle, stridor and stertor will all be reported as wheeze by parents
- There is no diagnostic test for childhood asthma but negative allergy tests may be useful in lowering the likelihood of an asthma diagnosis
- It may be appropriate to adopt a 'wait-and-see' policy or 2-month trial of low dose inhaled steroids in equivocal cases
- Chronic respiratory problems are common in children and are usually not due to asthma, especially in children aged under 2 years.

10.1 Introduction

There is no definitive test for asthma and this can make diagnosis difficult. This is especially true for the young child presenting with recurrent 'chestiness', i.e. cough and noisy breathing. The diagnosis lies in the history, since clinical examination is invariably normal.

10.2 History

Asthma is a chronic condition characterized by episodic wheeze, cough and shortness of breath. The clinician should elicit a history of these symptoms separated by symptom-free intervals. All children cough from time to time, so cough is not specific to asthma, and wheeze is therefore the cardinal symptom. 'Wheeze' is a term used by parents to describe a range of respiratory noise and it is therefore critical to establish what is actually meant by this term. Children with large airway rattle, stridor (sometimes due to croup) and stertor (sometimes due to adenoidal hypertrophy) are all said to 'wheeze'. Moreover, 75% of parents reporting wheeze in their preschool child will further characterize the sound as a rattle rather than a whistling noise. The simplest question to qualify reported wheeze is to ask 'is the sound a loud rattling sound or a soft whistling sound?'

In some consultations it is not possible to characterize the 'wheeze'. In such cases, it can be useful to ask whether the child was short of breath at the time when the noise was being made. The airway obstruction which causes wheeze will often cause an increase in respiratory rate and effort which is proportionate to the obstruction.

An alternative approach to clarifying the nature of noisy breathing is to ask the parent where the noise comes from; stertor comes from the nose, stridor and rattle from the throat and wheeze from the chest. Once a history of wheeze has been elicited, the final question to confirm the diagnosis is 'can the wheeze be brought on by a 'cold' and other triggers such as exercise, exposure to dogs, cold weather?'. Figure 10.1 summarizes the algorithm for diagnosing asthma in children.

There are further clues in the history in addition to the presence of episodic wheeze associated with cough and shortness of breath. Symptoms can be mild, moderate or severe (contrast with viral induced wheeze where symptoms are usually only moderate to severe). A first degree family history of asthma (parents and/ or siblings) increases the likelihood of asthma. Furthermore, a clear history of symptoms on exposure to cat, dog, grass or nuts is very suggestive of asthma (but such a clear history is not common). Coexisting allergic conditions, e.g. eczema, hay fever, and food allergies, modestly increase the probability of a child having asthma however it is important to remember that 75% of children with eczema do not have asthma (see Chapter 9).

Situations where asthma is not likely are those where there is only one symptom such as cough, wheeze or shortness of breath. Asthma is also less likely when the particular symptom is present all the time, when symptoms do not affect the child's quality of life, e.g. sleeping, exercise, or when the child has failure to thrive (Table 10.1).

Table 10.1 Clinical presentations that might be mistaken for childhood asthma

Presentation	Diagnoses	Clinical findings	Clinical Management
Wet cough in preschool child (particularly at night)	Bacterial bronchitis (very common)	Well thriving child, wet cough, no crackles/wheeze	Reassure
	Foreign body (less common)	Well child, often no history in inhalation, sudden onset cough without runny nose	Refer to specialist for diagnosis and treatment
	Cystic fibrosis (very rare)	Malnourished child, abdominal distention, +/– basal crackles	
	Ciliary dyskinesia (very rare)	Well child, recurrent middle ear disease, dextrocardia	
Episodic cough in school aged child	Pertussis	Normal out with coughing paroxysms, may have conjunctival haematoma	Macrolide if symptomatic for less than three weeks to prevent transmission. Advise cough will last 3–4 months
	Habitual cough (common)	Single loud cough only by day, often associated with anxiety	Reassure
Constant noisy breathing in infant/toddler	Rattle (or 'ruttle')	Course, monophonic inspiratory and expiratory sound ('Darth Vader'), palpable fremitus (chest felt to 'purr')	
	'Floppy airway' Laryngomalacia (common) Tracheo/bronchomalacia (less common)	Loud 'honking' cough, loud musical 'reed-like' noise on inspiration	Reassure if very young, feeding and thriving. If constantly present in child aged over one year refer to specialist for diagnosis and treatment
Episodic noisy breathing in school-aged child	Vocal cord disfunction	Terrifying episodes of inability to breath in, loud stridor, associated with exercise	Reassure, refer to breathing training

In some cases, particularly in young children, the diagnosis is not clear. In these instances a wait-and-see policy is appropriate if the child is thriving and otherwise well; alternatively a two month trial of low dose ICSs can be started. In a child with no evidence of failure to thrive and where symptoms have a minimal impact on the child's quality of life, neither of these options carries a particularly high risk. The evidence is that early treatment with ICSs does not alter the natural history of early onset asthma, in other words, early treatment does not make asthma less severe in future.

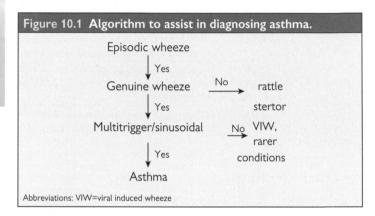

Figure 10.1 Algorithm to assist in diagnosing asthma.

Episodic wheeze

↓ Yes

Genuine wheeze — No → rattle

↓ Yes   stertor

Multitrigger/sinusoidal — No → VIW, rarer

↓ Yes   conditions

Asthma

Abbreviations: VIW=viral induced wheeze

10.3 **Physiological testing**

There is no test with acceptable sensitivity and specificity for asthma in children. Most asthmatic children will have normal spirometry (although this test is unable to adequately detect obstruction in small airways). Peak flow variability, skin prick testing, airway challenges and exhaled nitric oxide testing all lack sensitivity and specificity for asthma. However, lack of a positive allergy test and normal airway challenge/low exhaled nitric oxide may be useful in lowering the probability of asthma in a child with persistent respiratory symptoms. When weighing up the likelihood of asthma in children, greatest weight should always be placed on history; testing (if performed) should be undertaken to support the clinical suspicion.

10.4 **Viral induced wheeze**

The only common differential diagnosis for asthma is viral induced wheeze (also known as acute episodic wheeze). Viral induced wheeze can occur in children aged 6 months to 5 years (but can continue into later childhood) and is characterized by acute episodes of wheeze, cough and shortness of breath when the child has an (usually rhinovirus-induced) upper respiratory tract infection with rhinorrhoea. When the child is free of 'the cold' they have absolutely no symptoms. This 'all-or-nothing', 'on-or-off' pattern of symptoms is very different to the usual pattern of asthma where children can have mild, moderate or severe symptoms with and without rhinorrhoea. Additionally, viral induced wheeze is not associated with the airway eosinophilia seen in asthma and tends not to respond to treatment with oral or inhaled steroids. Inevitably the line of distinction between viral induced wheeze and asthma is not clear. At 3–4 years of age, some children with viral induced wheeze start wheezing without a cold and symptoms become less severe and asthma can often be diagnosed at that point. Some children cease wheezing but there is some evidence that these individuals will develop COPD in later life. The purpose of distinguishing between asthma and viral induced wheeze is that the former responds to ICS steroids whereas the latter generally does not, both respond to bronchodilators.

Further reading

Brand PL, Baraldi E, Bisgaard H, Boner AL, Castro-Rodriguez JA, Custovic A, et al. (2008) Definition, assessment and treatment of wheezing disorders in preschool children: an evidence-based approach. *Eur Respir J* **32**: 1096–110.

British Thoracic Society/Scottish Intercollegiate Guidelines Network (http://www.sign.ac.uk/guidelines/fulltext/101/index.html).

Global Initiative for Asthma (http://www.gina.org).

Chapter 11

Paediatric asthma: acute management

Steve Turner

> **Key points**
> - Acute asthma exacerbations are common in children
> - Most exacerbations are precipitated by viral upper respiratory tract infections, often in combination with other exposures
> - Assessment of severity is on clinical grounds
> - 25% of children admitted to hospital with acute asthma will be readmitted within 12 months and this can be reduced by good discharge planning.

11.1 Epidemiology

Acute childhood asthma remains a common and sometimes serious condition. In primary care, approximately 0.1% of all children attend each month due to acute asthma symptoms and the proportion is higher (0.6% in one study) in 5–14 year olds. The proportion of children presenting to primary care with acute asthma fell by approximately 25% between 1993 and 1998 and this is partly explained by improved asthma management and possibly also by falling asthma prevalence. In 2010, over 24,000 children were admitted to hospitals across England and Wales with acute asthma; the numbers treated in accident and emergency departments can be expected to be even greater. The proportion of children admitted with asthma relative to all admissions fell slightly between 1998 and 2004 from 19/1,000 to 17/1,000 admissions. Fortunately, deaths from acute asthma are uncommon in children and are also falling. Asthma mortality fell by approximately 70% between 1968 and 2000 but remains highest in 11–16 year olds. Between 1968 and 2000, asthma mortality (per 100,000 children/year) fell from 0.6 to 0.1 in 1–5 year olds, from 0.5 to 0.2 in 6–10 year olds and from 1.4 to 0.4 in 11–16 year olds.

Asthma exacerbations occur all year round but, in the northern hemisphere, there is an annual peak in asthma exacerbations in September.

11.2 **Aetiology**

Precipitants for acute asthma symptoms in children include viral upper respiratory tract infections, change in the weather, poor air quality, allergen exposure and exercise. Approximately 80% of childhood asthma exacerbations in primary care are associated with viral upper respiratory tract infections, predominantly due to rhinovirus (the common cold virus). The annual September 'epidemic' of exacerbations is mostly explained by rhinovirus infection which is spread through the community, probably due to people returning from summer holidays with rhinovirus strains which are new to their community. Changes in outdoor air quality, e.g. increasing concentrations of fine particulates, ozone, sulphur dioxide and oxides of nitrogen, are associated with increased presentation of children with acute asthma to emergency departments. Exposure to allergens which include house dust mite, cat and dog dander and grasses are also associated with increased risk for acute asthma exacerbation. Not every upper respiratory tract infection or exposure to poor air quality or allergen leads to an exacerbation. What is increasingly apparent is that interactions between exposures occur such that a child with asthma who has a 'cold' and exposed to allergen is more likely to have an exacerbation compared to a child exposed either to a 'cold' or allergen.

11.3 **Diagnosis**

Asthma is a recurrent condition and therefore acute asthma cannot be diagnosed on first presentation. For children presenting with their first episode of acute wheeze other conditions should be considered in addition to asthma. These include infection or aspiration of a foreign body. For children with a past history of acute wheeze, it is good clinical practice to establish the diagnosis of asthma and not merely presume that the child is a 'known asthmatic.' This is especially true in preschool children where the diagnosis is often less clear cut. A diagnosis of acute asthma should be applied with great caution in children under 2 years old. A child with a past history consistent with asthma who presents with asthma-like symptoms can be presumed to have asthma and not a lower respiratory tract infection.

11.4 **Assessment**

For the great majority of presentations, assessment is purely clinical and investigations such as blood gas analysis and chest x-ray should be sought only under exceptional circumstances. As for most paediatric presentations, clinical assessment of the child with acute asthma requires knowledge of age-appropriate normal values (Table 11.1). Historically, pulsus paradoxus (where the pulse volume falls during inspiration) was used as an index of assessment but this is no longer recommended.

11.5 **Management**

Management is dependent on (i) the assessment of severity and (ii) the assessment of response to treatment. The aim of management is to maintain oxygen saturations above 94%. In mild and moderate exacerbations, bronchodilators should only be administered via MDI/spacer combination. An MDI/spacer combination can be used in severe presentations but nebulizers can be more effective and offer the additional benefit of bronchodilator absorption across the buccal mucosa. Oral corticosteroids should be considered in all acute asthma. Intravenous corticosteroids should only be considered if the child is vomiting or has reduced consciousness (in the latter instance the priority should be maintaining airway and breathing and not corticosteroids). Intravenous treatment with salbutamol, aminophylline and magnesium sulphate (unlicensed indication) should be reserved for severe exacerbations where bronchodilators do not immediately reverse airway obstruction. There is no evidence that antibiotics should be used in the management of acute asthma exacerbations in children. All doses subsequently cited should be verified with local guidelines since there may be minor differences.

11.5.1 **Mild and moderate exacerbations**

Immediate treatment includes inhaled β_2-agonist via MDI/spacer combination, e.g. 2–10 puffs of salbutamol. A 3 day treatment with oral prednisolone (20 mg for children aged 2–5 years and 2 mg/kg up to a maximum of 40 mg for older children) should also usually be strongly considered.

11.5.2 **Severe exacerbations**

After supplemental oxygen has been applied, nebulized β_2-agonists (e.g. salbutamol) and muscarinic antagonists (e.g. ipratropium bromide) should be given in combination, since there is synergy between these therapies. Most guidelines suggest 5 mg nebulized

Table 11.1 Features associated with mild, moderate, severe or life-threatening exacerbation of asthma

		Respiratory rate (breaths/minute)	Pulse rate (beats/minute)	Respiratory effort	Oxygen saturations	Other clinical features
Mild	2–5 years	<30	<120	Normal	>95%	Soft wheeze
	5–11 years	<20	<100			
	>11 years	<15	<90			
Moderate	2–5 years	30–40	120–140	Some recession	92–95%	Obvious wheeze
	5–11 years	20–30	100–125	Some use of accessory muscles		Obvious wheeze, talks in phrases, prefers to sit rather than lie, %PEF 50–75%*
	>11 years	15–25	90–11			
Severe	2–5 years	>40	>140	Obvious recession	<92%	Difficulty drinking
	5–11 years	>30	>125	Obvious use of accessory muscles		Talks in words %PEF 33–50*, agitated, sits hunched forward
	>11 years	≥25	≥110			
Life-threatening	2–5 years	As for severe asthma				Visibly cyanosed, silent chest, reduced consciousness, poor respiratory effort
	5–11 years					
	>11 years					

*%PEF = percentage of predicted PEF

salbutamol every 20 minutes over an hour with the first dose combined with 250 micrograms of ipratropium bromide. In those who do not respond to nebulized treatment, additional treatment with intravenous salbutamol should be considered (15 micrograms/kg over 10 minutes) and or a single bolus of intravenous magnesium sulphate (1–2 grammes) (unlicensed indication). Intravenous aminophylline has been proven to be effective in the past but appears to be no more effective than intravenous salbutamol but with more side effects—in particular nausea—and requires plasma levels to be checked after 24 hours.

11.5.3 Life threatening exacerbations

These are rare but require prompt recognition and management. Treatment with nebulized and intravenous bronchodilators should be commenced and senior medical and anaesthetic support sought urgently.

11.6 Discharge planning

Approximately 25% of children admitted to hospital with acute asthma will be readmitted within the following year. This proportion was reduced to 8% in a study where a nurse-led educational intervention was used. Asthma admissions are associated with poor understanding of treatment, poor compliance and poor inhaler technique. The discharge process should address these issues and include education, motivation and assessment of inhaler technique. Children and parents should be given an action plan on discharge and ideally a medical review within the following 30 days.

11.7 Preventing future asthma exacerbations

Other than good discharge planning, there is little evidence for other interventions which reduce the risk or severity of future asthma exacerbations. In a study funded by the pharmaceutical industry, additional treatment with a LTRA between September and mid-October was shown to reduce symptoms during the annual epidemic. There is also evidence that parent-initiated treatment with oral prednisolone, compared to clinician-initiated treatment, is associated with (surprisingly) minor improvements in symptoms during exacerbations. Although often recommended, there is no evidence that increasing dose of ICS during an exacerbation is beneficial.

Further reading

British Thoracic Society/Scottish Intercollegiate Guidelines Network (http://www.sign.ac.uk/guidelines/fulltext/101/index.html).

Global Initiative for Asthma (http://www.gina.org).

Johnston SL, Pattemore PK, Sanderson G, Smith S, Lampe F, Josephs L, et al. (1995) Community study of role of viral infections in exacerbations of asthma in 9–11 year old children. Brit Med J **310**: 1225–9.

Madge P, McColl J, Paton J (1997) Impact of a nurse-led home management training programme in children admitted to hospital with acute asthma: a randomised controlled study. Thorax **52**: 223–8.

Ordonez GA, Phelan PD, Olinsky A, Robertson CF (1998) Preventable factors in hospital admissions for asthma. Arch Dis Child **78**: 143–7.

Panickar JR, Dodd SR, Smyth RL, Couriel JM (2005) Trends in deaths from respiratory illness in children in England and Wales from 1968 to 2000. Thorax **60**: 1035–8.

Chapter 12

Paediatric asthma: chronic management

Steve Turner

> **Key points**
> - Asthma control is measured by symptom scores and not PEF or spirometry
> - Spending time with children and parents on an asthma management plan is important
> - Low dose ICS control asthma symptoms in the vast majority of children
> - In children with poor asthma control despite low dose ICSs, the diagnosis should be reconsidered, non-compliance explored and inhaler technique assessed.

12.1 Overview

The goals of asthma management are to enable the child and their family to live a normal life. Due to the nature of the disease, management is driven by patient-reported symptoms. The step-up and step-down approach to asthma treatment has become widely accepted as good practice but treatment is only effective when the diagnosis is correct and drugs are taken correctly.

12.2 Asthma control

Historically, asthma treatment has been driven by the severity of symptoms. More recently, clinicians have recognized that good overall control is a more appropriate target since a severe asthmatic can have well-controlled symptoms while a mild asthmatic can have poorly-controlled symptoms. Well-controlled asthma is characterized by no day-to-day symptoms and no exacerbations (Box 12.1);

Box 12.1 Goals of asthma control

- Prevent chronic and troublesome symptoms
- Reduce the need for as required bronchodilators (i.e. use on 0, 1, or 2 days a week)
- Maintain normal activity level and undisturbed sleep
- Prevent asthma exacerbations.
- Maintain good lung function

poor day-to-day asthma control is a good predictor of future exacerbations. The key to good control in the short and long term is therefore 'keeping on top' of daily symptoms.

The Children's Asthma Control Test (http://www.asthmacontroltest.com/children.htm) is one of a number of tools by which overall asthma control can be assessed.

To achieve good asthma control, all children should have a management plan where the child's goals are described. Some examples of child-centred goals are listed in Box 12.2. Management is more likely to be successful when the child and parent are actively involved in the goal setting process. Ideally there are green, amber and red areas where symptoms trigger changes in management.

Box 12.2 Examples of child-centred goals of asthma control

- I can play football without stopping for an inhaler
- I can ride a horse without wheezing
- I can play outside at school break time during winter
- I will not to be admitted to hospital before my next birthday
- I can go to sleep-overs and not wake my friends with coughing.

In the past, PEF measurements have figured highly in asthma management plans but much less emphasis (if any) should be placed on these measurements due to their poor sensitivity and specificity for the population as a whole. Anecdotally, there are children in whom peak flow measurements are usefully linked with symptoms but these represent a minority.

12.3 **Therapeutic treatment of childhood asthma**

The step-up step-down approach (Figure 12.1) to asthma treatment has been adopted by most guidelines and reflects the typical relapse/remission pattern of asthma symptoms over time.

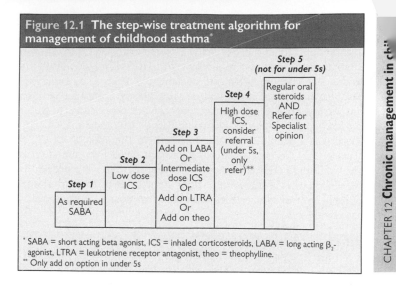

Figure 12.1 The step-wise treatment algorithm for management of childhood asthma*

Step 1
As required SABA

Step 2
Low dose ICS

Step 3
Add on LABA
Or
Intermediate dose ICS
Or
Add on LTRA
Or
Add on theo

Step 4
High dose ICS, consider referral (under 5s, only refer)**

Step 5
(not for under 5s)
Regular oral steroids
AND
Refer for Specialist opinion

* SABA = short acting beta agonist, ICS = inhaled corticosteroids, LABA = long acting β_2-agonist, LTRA = leukotriene receptor antagonist, theo = theophylline.
** Only add on option in under 5s

12.3.1 **Step one: as required SABAs**

These include drugs such as salbutamol and terbutaline both of which act at the β_2 adrenoceptor in the airways. This class of drug is very effective for relief of acute symptoms. Some children continue to be wrongly advised to take SABA twice a day regardless of symptoms; regular treatment may render some children relatively insensitive to SABA treatment during exacerbations. One sixth of the population have a genetic variant of the β_2 adrenoceptor which causes regular treatment to reduce the number of receptors being expressed by cells and in this context when the child becomes ill, bronchodilators may not be as effective.

Requirement for SABA for more than two days a week is an indication that asthma is not well controlled and preventers should be considered. Muscarinic receptor antagonists, e.g. ipratropium bromide, have bronchodilator properties but are not indicated for childhood asthma unless nebulized in combination with a SABA in cases of acute severe asthma (see Chapter 11).

12.3.2 **Step two: start low dose ICS**

Asthma is a very steroid-sensitive condition in children and the majority of patients will respond to low dose treatment (i.e. 200 micrograms budesonide or 100 micrograms fluticasone per day for children under 12 years old). Treatment is only effective when taken and the degree of compliance should be explored and optimised before increasing beyond step two.

12.3.3 Step three: start non-steroidal add-on or increase ICS

In adult populations there is clearly a benefit in adding LABAs to step 2 treatments compared to increasing the ICS dose. However, the evidence in children is less well documented. A study by Lemanske *et al.* demonstrated that children with poorly controlled asthma despite low dose ICS respond in roughly equal proportions to either the addition of LABA or increasing ICS or the addition of LTRA; there was a marginally greater response to the addition of LABA (Figure 12.2). Perhaps an equally important result from this study is that whilst 182 children took part in the study, 128 were previously excluded from the study due to poor compliance or their symptoms became controlled once they took their low dose ICS treatment.

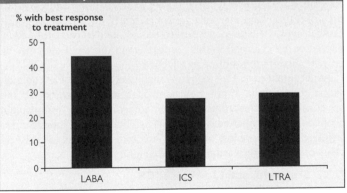

Figure 12.2 Bar charts from study by Lemanske *et al.* demonstrating which step 3 treatment option was associated with 'best response' to treatment. In random order, children aged 6 to 17 years received 16 weeks of each of the three treatment options. Best response was determined by need for oral steroid for exacerbation, daily symptom score and lung function. From *N Engl J Med*, Lemanske RFJ, Mauger DT, Sorkness CA, et al. , Step up therapy for children with uncontrolled asthma while receiving inhaled corticosteroids, 362:975–985. Copyright © (2010) Massachusetts Medical Society. Reprinted with permission from Massachusetts Medical Society.

The consensus is that LABA should be added before ICS dose is increased to an intermediate dose (i.e. 400 micrograms/day budesonide or 200 micrograms day fluticasone for children aged under 12 years). LABA should never be prescribed without ICS due to the potential for down regulation of beta 2 adrenoreceptors as described in step 1 above. If the addition of LABA or an increase to an intermediate dose of ICS do not control symptoms, then a LTRA, e.g. monteleukast, should be added to low dose ICS. Finally theophylline can be added. While steps 1, 2, 4 and 5 are straight forward, step 3 is more complex and reflects the lack of evidence suggesting that any of the four options is clearly superior.

12.3.4 Step four: start high dose ICS in children 5–12 years old

If the treatment options in step 3 do not control symptoms in children aged 5–12 years, high dose ICS should be started (i.e. 800 micrograms/day budesonide or 500 micrograms/day fluticasone). There is evidence that for the population as a whole, a ceiling effect exists where ICS doses above 400 micrograms do not improve asthma control. However, there are some individuals in whom increasing to high doses is associated with improved asthma control, and this remains an important treatment option. What is also understood is that ICS side-effects are more common at higher doses. The dose-response relationship between ICS and treatment effects is not linear and is shown in Figure 12.3. For children aged under five years, the management of asthma not responding to step 3 treatments for children is simple: do not use high dose ICS or oral steroids but refer for urgent specialist opinion.

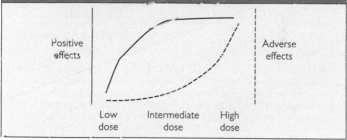

Figure 12.3 Schematic diagram illustrating the flattening of the dose response relationship between higher doses of ICS and beneficial outcomes (solid lines) and the rising relationship between adverse effects (broken lines) as higher doses are used

12.3.5 Step five: start regular oral steroids

This is an extremely uncommon step to take and arguably should only be made by a specialist clinician once the diagnosis is confirmed beyond reasonable doubt, compliance is confirmed and psychological issues are identified and addressed (see when treatment does not work).

12.4 **Different treatments for different age-groups**

Across the paediatric age range there are three different treatment algorithms and for this reason children can be over- or under-treated. Differences are outlined in Box 12.3.

Box 12.3 Differences in treatment options and doses for children at different ages.

- **Under 5 years old:** Step 2 includes either low dose ICS or LTRA. There is no indication for LABA or theophylline in this age range. At step 3, the dose of ICS can be increased to intermediate dose and LTRA added. Young children failing to respond to step 3 treatment should be referred for specialist opinion without treatment being further escalated

- **5 to 12 years old:** These treatment steps are shown in figure 12.1.

- **Over 12 years old:** These children are considered adults and low dose of daily ICS for this age-range is 200–800 micrograms with the suggested starting dose being 400 micrograms/day for step 2. For step 3 the ceiling dose of ICS remains 800 micrograms/day and LABA should be added. For step 4, the ceiling dose of ICS increases to 2000 micrograms/day and an oral beta agonist tablet can be prescribed in addition to oral LTRA and theophylline. Step 5 is the addition of oral steroid.

12.5 **When does treatment not work?**

Childhood asthma is invariably sensitive to low dose ICS but in some individuals, treatment above step 2 is required. When children reach treatment steps 3, 4, and 5, the following scenarios should be considered:

1. The diagnosis is wrong. This is more common in younger children (see chapter 10).

2. The medication is not being taken. Compliance with inhaled medication in children is conservatively estimated at no more than 50% and closer to 70% for oral medication. Assessment of compliance can be challenging, although determining the number of prescriptions for preventers which have been requested (should be approximately one inhaler per month) may give insight into how much preventer is being used. Compliance can be improved in children prescribed ICS and LABA by using a combination inhaler (i.e. an inhaler containing both medications).

3. The inhaled medication is not being taken correctly. See inhaler devices (Section 12.7).
4. There is ongoing exposure to an environmental factor. Such factors might include second hand tobacco smoke or animal dander. Whilst there is evidence that asthma control improves with reduced exposure to products of tobacco smoke, there is very little evidence that allergen avoidance in the home improves asthma control.
5. There are behavioural elements to the illness. It can be challenging to separate anxiety about asthma symptoms from apparent asthma symptoms due to anxiety (somatization). Suggestive features include: requirement for very frequent use of SABA (e.g. exhausting one SABA canister in a week) despite a history of few, brief hospitalizations with asthma; low self-esteem; other features of anxiety (e.g. school avoidance); contemporaneous social disruption (e.g. parental separation). A psychologist opinion may be helpful but, ultimately, it is the clinician who has to decide how much of the reported symptoms are due to asthma and how much are due to anxiety.
6. There is genuinely severe asthma. Whilst steroid-resistant asthma is described in adults, this phenomenon is not reported in children but this possibility should be considered when points 1–5 above have been considered and addressed. In this setting, there may be an indication for carefully supervised trials conducted in specialist centres of medications such as anti-IgE antibody (olamizumab), ciclosporin or continuous subcutaneous SABA infusion.

12.6 **Stepping down and stopping treatment**

There are two possible explanations for symptoms being well-controlled on medication: first asthma has gone into remission and second the treatment is palliating the underlying asthma. Stepping down preventative treatment, or stopping if on step 2, carries an inherent risk of unmasking symptoms and there is no test which can aid this clinical decision. The consensus is that treatment should be stepped down, or stopped if on step 2, if symptoms have been controlled for 3 months.

12.7 **Inhaler devices**

Inhaled asthma medications can be delivered by one of four methods: MDI, breath actuated inhaler, dry powder device and nebulizer. A MDI should never be given to a child without a spacer device.

n adult's small airways receive approximately 5% of the drug delivered by an MDI without a spacer and this tiny proportion is lower in children. In contrast, an MDI with spacer will deliver approximately 20% of the drug to the smaller airways. An MDI must be shaken before each puff; failure to do this will halve the amount of drug delivered. A spacer gathers static charge and this can double retention of drug in the spacer; rinsing in warm soapy water once a month effectively removes static charge from a spacer. The most common explanation for an MDI/spacer combination to fail to work is not shaking the MDI and not to remove static charge. Although licensed for use in children aged 5 years and above, dry powder and breath actuated devices are often not suitable for children under 8 years of age since young children often cannot generate at the required inspiratory flows.

A common reason for dry powder or breath actuated devices failing to control symptoms is failure to deliver drug to the small airways and an MDI/spacer combination should be considered. There is no role for nebulizers in the routine management of asthma in children.

12.8 **Side effects of asthma treatment**

At prescribed doses, there are no serious side effects associated with asthma treatment. Children prescribed ICS may experience a reduction in growth velocity of 1 cm for the first year but thereafter growth is not affected. High dose, off label ICS doses are associated with adrenocortical suppression which sadly has been associated with fatality. Short or long synacthen tests can be used to monitor adrenal suppression but the relationship between dose of ICS and cortical suppression is extremely heterogeneous; most children receiving high dose ICS do not have adrenal suppression whereas a small, idiosyncratic minority on conventional ICS doses have features of adrenal suppression (i.e. non-specific lethargy, muscle aches, early morning hypoglycaemia). Parents and children in receipt of high dose ICS should be alerted to the symptoms of adrenal suppression and issued with a steroid warning card.

12.9 **Non-therapeutic management of childhood asthma**

The management of childhood asthma is not solely based on prescribing medications. Good management includes spending time with children and parents to agree the asthma management plan, assessing inhaler technique, planning for exacerbations and addressing obvious environmental precipitants. Although much store is conventionally set by reduced allergen exposure (in particular laminate flooring, removing feather bedding, and special vacuum cleaners) there is no evidence to support this activity since the interventions do not alter the burden of domestic allergen. There is good evidence that children with asthma who are very allergic to a single allergen, e.g. grass, will benefit from immunotherapy, i.e. exposure to high concentrations of allergen. This treatment should only be delivered in specialist centres.

At least 40% of children with asthma are exposed to second hand tobacco smoke and 5% of adolescents with asthma are regular smokers; these exposures should therefore be addressed. There is no evidence that humidifiers, dehumidifiers or atomizers improve asthma control. Similarly, there is no evidence that weight loss improves asthma control but all overweight and obese children should be encouraged to take smaller sized portions and exercise regularly. Although the flu vaccine is recommended for children with asthma and that this effectively prevents flu, there is little evidence that the influenza virus causes asthma exacerbations.

Further reading

Asthma (children under 5)—inhaler devices, NICE guideline (http://egap. evidence.nhs.uk/TA10).

British Thoracic Society/Scottish Intercollegiate Guidelines Network (http://www. sign.ac.uk/guidelines/fulltext/101/index.html).

Glasgow NJ, Ponsonby A-L, Kemp A, Tovey E, van Asperen P, McKay K, Forbes S (2011) Feather bedding and childhood asthma associated with house dust mite sensitisation: a randomised controlled trial. *Arch Dis Child* **96**: 541–7.

Global Initiative for Asthma (http://www.gina.org).

Lemanske RFJ, Mauger DT, Sorkness CA, *et al.* (2010) Step up therapy for children with uncontrolled asthma while receiving inhaled corticosteroids. *N Engl J Med* DOI: 10.1056/NEJMoa1001278.

Chapter 13

Asthma in primary care

Cathy M. Jackson

> **Key points**
>
> - The primary care contract recognizes that the responsibility for the diagnosis and long-term management of asthma lies principally with the primary healthcare team
> - Overall outcomes are best when doctors and nurses trained in asthma deliver the service in primary care
> - The Quality Outcome Framework (QOF) of the primary care contract in the UK sets out four revised indicators of quality of care of patients with asthma
> - Review should be proactive rather than reactive.

13.1 **The primary care contract**

The UK primary care contract recognizes asthma as a common condition in which responsibility for both the diagnosis and subsequent long-term management lies principally with the primary healthcare team. Indeed, asthma is one of the most common chronic conditions diagnosed in a primary care setting. The majority of all asthmatics will be managed entirely by the primary team with secondary care referral occurring in only a small minority of more challenging cases.

To ensure that the quality of care provided for all patients with asthma is optimal, it is important to have in place mechanisms for identifying these patients, ensuring regular review and employing staff capable of delivering current best practice. While most practices have had some form of asthma clinic in place for many years, the QOF of the UK general practice contract has necessitated that information on all patients is complete and readily accessible. This has led to many healthcare teams reviewing and improving the consistency of delivery of care. The current British Thoracic Society/ Scottish Intercollegiate Guidelines Network (BTS/SIGN) guidelines for the management of asthma advise primary care teams to audit their asthma caseload and tailor the care they deliver to the particular needs of their practice.

Asthma lends itself to assessment of quality of care by outcome. This is largely due to it being an area where there are widely accepted clinical guidelines and good evidence to suggest that, in the populations studied, health benefits can be achieved if there are mechanisms in place to ensure that guidelines are followed in practice. The revised QOF of the primary care contract currently sets out only four indicators of quality of care of patients with asthma (Table 13.1), which in turn determines the level of payment received for provision of that care. Previous versions of QOF have had larger numbers of indicators for asthma but as several of these have now become accepted everyday practice, the need for the financial incentives of the QOF has been removed.

Table 13.1 Revised QOF for asthma for primary care contract	
Records	'The practice can produce a register of patients with asthma, excluding patients with asthma who have been prescribed no asthma-related drugs in the last 12 months'
Initial management	'The percentage of patients aged eight and over diagnosed as having asthma from 1 April 2006 with measures of variability or reversibility'
Continuing management	'The percentage of patients with asthma between the ages of 14 and 19 in whom there is a record of smoking status in the previous 15 months'
Continuing management	'The percentage of patients with asthma who have had an asthma review in the last 15 months'

This set of indicators was developed in line with the BTS/SIGN guidelines, although it provides only a very crude measurement of the quality level for provision of care. The requirement for this information to guide the level of payment received has ensured that all practices revisit the manner in which they deliver care and where necessary, changes are made to current practice to ensure a consistently high level of care.

13.2 Diagnosis

As asthma is most commonly diagnosed in primary care, the first step in the provision of care is the ability to diagnose it with a degree of confidence. Symptoms may vary widely between individuals, and the disease may become quiescent for long periods of time. Active inflammation of the airways can also be present without the patient being aware of any symptoms. These three factors can make both the diagnosis and management of asthma challenging at times.

The diagnosis is most frequently made on the basis of the history with supporting evidence from lung function tests (see Chapter 2). QOF indicators also suggest that this should be accompanied by recordings of variability and/or reversibility. During history taking, it is important not only to consider the nature, timing and duration of symptoms but also family history, smoking, occupation, recreational activities, pets, known allergies, current medication and identify the presence or absence of symptoms of rhinitis and atopy.

13.3 Management

The detailed management of chronic asthma is detailed in Chapter 4. In acute asthma, a guide to management in primary care (and when to refer to hospital) is shown in Figure 13.1.

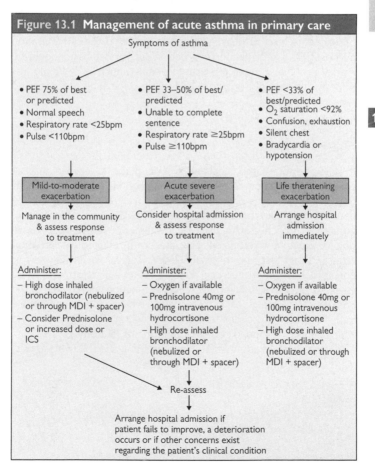

Figure 13.1 Management of acute asthma in primary care

13.4 **Reasons for referral**

It is occasionally necessary to refer patients for further investigations or management decisions. Patients requiring a further opinion might include those for whom there is doubt about the diagnosis and may require further investigations, those who remain symptomatic or have frequent exacerbations despite being at step 3 on the BTS/SIGN guidelines. It is also reasonable to refer patients whose current or previous occupation may play a part in symptoms in order to accurately assess their condition and any causative agents.

13.5 **Recording**

Once confident of the diagnosis of asthma, patient details should be recorded in a regularly updated, and preferably electronic and password protected, disease register of all cases. This should ideally include all relevant information for ongoing management and demonstrate the level of quality outcomes achieved for remuneration purposes. The information recorded in such a database should be readily retrievable using any search enquiry, such as '>12 months since last review', not only for QOF but also for audit purposes and service planning.

13.6 **Review**

It is important that a mechanism is in place to ensure that all patients with asthma are offered the opportunity to have their condition reviewed on a regular basis with a frequency determined by need—but at least once every 12 months. Current evidence suggests that 'proactive structured review, as opposed to opportunistic or unscheduled review, is associated with reduced exacerbation rates and days lost from normal activity'. Regular review allows not only patient's symptoms, lung function tests and treatment to be assessed, but can also fulfill several other functions. A key role of the primary care professional is to recognize which patients need more frequent reviews in order to maximize their symptom control and which patients will need review appointments less often.

As a basic minimum, the QOF suggests that the following assessment is carried out at review appointments:

• Assess symptoms using the Royal College of Physicians' three questions:
  1. In the last month have you had difficulty sleeping because of your asthma symptoms (including cough)?

2. In the last month have you had your usual asthma symptoms during the day (cough, wheeze, chest tightness or breathlessness)?

3. In the last month has your asthma interfered with your usual activities, e.g. housework, work/school, etc.?

- PEF value
- Inhaler technique
- Ensuring that individuals have a personalized asthma plan.

If asthma appears to be uncontrolled the QOF suggests that the following should also be examined as part of the review before adjusting treatment:

- Smoking behaviour
- Inhaler technique
- Concordance with regular preventative therapy
- Identification of symptoms suggestive of rhinitis.

A review appointment also facilitates an opportunity to discuss with patients any anxieties regarding asthma in general, management regimes or problems that may affect the patient's ability to take treatment as prescribed. A review appointment can also provide an opportunity for patient education in terms of self-management, lifestyle factors and vaccination.

An individually tailored asthma management plan should be drawn up together with the patient thereby allowing them to have a greater degree of control over their own treatment (Box 13.1). This provides a straightforward means of monitoring peak flow recordings and can highlight to the patient and healthcare professionals involved in their care, any deterioration.

Box 13.1 Asthma Management Plan

- Asthma management plans have been shown to improve compliance and reduce delay in referral to hospital
- A good asthma management plan should:
  - Help the patient understand the nature of their disease
  - Detail the patient's regular medications
  - Advise them when to change/increase this medication
  - Suggest who to contact if symptoms get worse/fail to improve
  - Explain how and when to return to usual doses following an exacerbation
  - Indicate when urgent medical help is indicated.

Smoking status can also be checked and patients who smoke should also be assessed as to their readiness to quit and interventions offered where necessary. Perhaps one of the most useful functions of a regular review appointment is to strengthen the relationship and approachability between those providing the service and the patient. This may enable queries or concerns regarding the patient's condition or treatment to be addressed *before* problems are encountered.

13.7 **Staff development**

Since asthma is a common chronic disorder, ongoing staff training should be a priority for all practices. Indeed, good asthma management relies on all members of the primary care team having a suitable level of knowledge and ensuring that all individuals are not only trained in current best practice but are also able to access current guidelines and have the time and facilities to be able to apply them. Training should not only involve current treatment regimes and future treatments, but also encompass those communication skills likely to improve an individual's understanding of asthma and encourage concordance with treatment plans and changes in lifestyle where appropriate. Training should apply not only to clinical staff, but also administrative staff, to enable automatic recall of patients and recording and retrieval of data.

13.8 **Limitations of QOF**

At present the QOF uses only the revised criteria of: being able to identify asthmatics, the number diagnosed with a measure of variability and/or reversibility, those with a review within the last 15 months, and assessment of smoking status in young patients with asthma. These are considered to be the areas in which further work now needs to be done and builds on the previous indicators which laid the foundations for the very basic requirements of asthma management which aimed to ensure that every practice is able to provide a streamlined care plan for every patient.

The revised QOF indicators have included the suggestion that the presence of rhinitis should be enquired about if asthma control has yet to be achieved Many patients with asthma experience symptoms from active rhinitis and current evidence and guidelines suggest that if upper airways inflammation is optimally treated, a commensurate improvement in asthma control will be achieved.

There is at present surprisingly little evidence that monitoring symptoms, PEF, inhaler technique and lifestyle in primary care will have any effect on the course of the disease in patients. At present, most research is performed in a secondary care setting, which represents individuals at the more severe extreme of the disease spectrum who are not truly reflective of the majority of patients with asthma. As a consequence, findings may not be applicable to the asthma population as a whole. Moreover, one unforeseen advantage of the new QOF data is that databases produced by practices may allow researchers to access information more easily. This, in turn, may increase the amount of evidence-based data and research produced from a primary care setting with the ultimate aim of improving the care of all patients with asthma.

Websites

Useful websites for clinicians:

- http://www.brit-thoracic.org.uk (British Thoracic Society)
- http://www.nhsemployers.org/PayAndContracts/
  GeneralMedicalServicesContract/QOF/Pages/
  QualityOutcomesFramework.aspx (accessed March 2011)
- http://www.pcrs-uk.org/ (Primary Care Respiratory Society)
- http://www.occupationalasthma.com (occupational asthma website)
- http://www.sign.ac.uk (Scottish Intercollegiate Guidelines Network).

Useful websites for patients:

- http://www.asthma.org.uk (leading UK asthma charity)
- http://www.allergyuk.org (UK allergy foundation)
- http://www.lunguk.org (leading UK lung charity)
- http://www.laia.ac.uk (Lung and Asthma Information Agency).

Further reading

Allergic Rhinitis and its Impact on Asthma (ARIA) guidelines: 2010 revision.

British Guideline on the Management of Asthma (2008) British Thoracic Society Scottish Intercollegiate Guidelines Network.*Thorax* **63**(4): iv1–121.

Brozek JL, Bousquet J, Baena-Cagnani CE, Bonini S, Canonica GW, Casale TB, van Wijk RG, Ohta K, Zuberbier T, Schünemann HJ (2010) Global Allergy and Asthma European Network; Grading of Recommendations Assessment, Development and Evaluation Working Group. *J Allergy Clin Immunol* **126**: 466–76.

Lindberg M, Ahlner J, Möller M, Ekström T (1999) Asthma nurse practice—a resource-effective approach in asthma management. *Respir Med* **93**: 584–8.

Chapter 14

Difficult asthma

Claire A. Butler and Liam G. Heaney

> **Key points**
>
> - Always consider whether patients do actually have asthma; consider further tests to help confirm the diagnosis if necessary
> - Consider whether patients may have a co-existent condition
> - Determine whether any aggravating factors may be present
> - Always ask about adherence to treatment
> - Consider checking blood theophylline, prednisolone or cortisol levels when indicated
> - Assess inhaler technique at every opportunity.

14.1 Introduction

Most patients with asthma respond to standard doses of ICSs with or without additional therapies such as LABAs, theophyllines or LTRAs. Effective treatment along with asthma action plans should mean that the majority of patients can expect minimal breakthrough symptoms on standard doses of treatment. However, a small group of patients present with persistent asthma symptoms despite effective therapy, and are often referred to as having 'difficult-to-control asthma'.

14.2 The 'difficult asthmatic'

A pragmatic definition of difficult asthma is persistent respiratory symptoms, despite treatment with a LABA and high dose ICSs (≥1000 ug beclometasone equivalent) and at least one course of rescue steroids in the preceding 12 months. This equates with subjects who remain symptomatic despite treatment at Global Initiative for Asthma step 4/5. It is estimated that between 5 and 10% of adult patients with asthma fulfil this definition, although the exact prevalence is uncertain.

A recent World Health Organization Consultation on severe asthma proposed three sub-groups of patients under the 'severe asthma' umbrella:

1. Untreated severe asthma
2. Difficult-to-treat severe asthma
3. Treatment-resistant severe asthma (patients who have high treatment requirements to control their disease).

Four components for assessment of asthma severity adapted from the NAEPP-EPR3 2007 (National Asthma Education and Prevention Program) have been suggested and includes level of control (encompassing current clinical control over the previous 2–4 weeks, exacerbations over the past 6–12 months and use of oral corticosteroids), current treatment requirements, response to treatment and risk (likelihood of asthma exacerbations and development of chronic morbidity).

The probability that patients with severe asthma are a heterogeneous group with the requirement for targeted—rather than blanket—therapy has led to interest in further phenotyping. A cluster analysis of asthma phenotypes from the Severe Asthma Research Program identified five groups of patients with severe asthma. These included:

1. Early-onset atopic asthma with normal lung function (2 or less controller medications)
2. Early-onset atopic asthma with preserved lung function (increase medication requirements)
3. Late-onset non-atopic asthma with reduction in FEV_1 (mostly older obese females)
4. Early-onset generally atopic asthma with severe but reversible reduction in FEV_1 (high medication use)
5. Early-onset less atopic asthma with severe and poorly reversible reduction in FEV_1 (high medication use and frequent rescue steroid use).

From an assessment and therapeutic perspective, it is important to differentiate the term 'difficult asthma' from 'therapy-resistant asthma' or 'refractory asthma'; the latter terms encompass patients who are relatively treatment resistant and require high doses of corticosteroids to achieve symptom control. In contrast, patients with 'difficult asthma' often have many different factors, which cause them to respond poorly to treatment. It is important to adopt a systematic approach to the assessment and management of this group of patients, and a number of key questions should be asked before committing them to further high and often prolonged courses of oral corticosteroids.

14.2.1 Does the patient have asthma?

When faced with a patient with difficult asthma who is not respond-ing to conventional therapy, it is important to confirm the diagnosis of asthma by reviewing the history and objective corroborative mea-sures of asthma, such as reversible airflow obstruction or airway hyperresponsiveness. If satisfied that the patient definitely has asthma, it is then important to identify other concomitant conditions, which may result in 'asthma-like' symptoms; these are often inappro-priately treated as asthma.

Alternative diagnoses are commonly identified after systematic evaluation—19% and 34% in the two published case series of difficult asthmatics (Table 14.1). When these conditions are correctly iden-tified and managed, this will generally lead to an improvement in symptom control, without escalating asthma therapy. It is important to re-emphasize that in many cases, these conditions and asthma co-exist; for example, around one-third of patients with vocal cord dys-function are thought to have asthma. Thus, many other conditions can cause asthma-like symptoms, and not surprisingly are associated with a poor response to asthma treatment. Identification and management of these should improve symptoms and allow a reduction of asthma medication.

Table 14.1 Alternative/concomitant diagnoses in difficult asthma

Alternative Condition	Diagnosis	Management
Bronchiectasis	Steroid-unresponsive, productive cough Recurrent bacterial infection with sputum purulence Typical HRCT findings	Training in mucus clearance techniques Antibiotic treatment of infections Maintenance macrolide therapy
Dysfunctional breathlessness/ Hyperventilation syndrome	Atypical symptoms and breathlessness out of keeping with lung function	Explanation Graded exercise program
COPD	Fixed airflow obstruction Exertional breathlessness unresponsive to increasing medication	Bronchodilators Pulmonary Rehabilitation
Vocal cord dysfunction	Inspiratory stridor when symptomatic (due to paradoxical inspiratory vocal cord adduction) Variable inspiratory and expiratory flow volume loops	Speech and language input Treatment of psychological co-morbidity

Other less common diagnoses may include chronic bronchitis, IgA deficiency, cystic fibrosis, obliterative bronchiolitis, cardiomyopathy, pulmonary hypertension, hypereosinophilia, extrinsic allergic alveolitis, respiratory muscle incoordination, and obstructive sleep apnoea.

14.2.2 **Are they taking their treatment?**

Poor adherence occurs throughout the spectrum of asthma severity and is an important reason for an apparent poor response to treatment. Both patient and physician reporting are recognized to be consistently unreliable and direct measurements such as plasma theophylline levels or plasma prednisolone and cortisol measurements are useful in this respect. Assessment of adherence to inhaled therapy is difficult, although surrogate measures such as prescription filling of maintenance inhalers can be useful. A recent study of non-adherence in a Difficult Asthmatic population of 182 patients found that 34% were collecting less than 50% of their prescribed inhalation medication. In addition, approximately 50% of patients on maintenance oral corticosteroid were found to be non-adherent when plasma prednisolone and cortisol levels were assessed in two separate case series of difficult asthmatics. Despite ongoing asthma symptoms, many patients choose not to take their treatment as prescribed and issues underlying non-adherence must be explored.

Poor adherence may result from a number of factors including fear of side-effects, lack of immediate effect following ICSs, poor education, resentment by adolescents about the need for therapy, economic restriction on access to health care, demographic factors such as sex and ethnicity and secondary gain from ongoing symptoms.

It can be difficult to question patients regarding poor adherence as this can lead to breakdown of the physician-patient relationship, and needs to be addressed in an empathetic and non-confrontational manner. The key issue is identifying the particular reason for non-adherence in an individual. Adequate education can allay any fears that a patient may have regarding their treatment, especially the potential side-effect of corticosteroids. A recent two-phase study by Gamble *et al.* reported increased adherence to prescribed inhaled combination therapy in addition to reduced daily ICS dose and requirement for rescue steroid courses following a nurse-led menu driven intervention. Thus, identification and intervention of non-adherence in this population can lead to improved outcome.

14.2.3 **Are there additional aggravating factors?**

It is important to identify other factors which may be driving asthma symptoms. These may include:

- Intrinsic factors
  - Psychological factors
  - Upper airways disease
  - Gastro-oesophageal reflux
  - Systemic disease (thyrotoxicosis, Churg-Strauss syndrome, carcinoid syndrome)
- Extrinsic factors
  - Drugs
  - Inhaled allergen exposure
  - Occupational factors.

There is a much debated link between asthma control and psychological stress. It is likely that difficult-to-control asthma results in considerable psychological stress for patients, especially if there has been a history of life-threatening exacerbations. However, it is also likely that psychological factors can worsen asthma control. Psychosocial morbidity has been associated with asthma death and near fatal asthma. In a Belfast study, psychiatric morbidity was common when formally assessed by a medical liaison psychiatrist, with 32 of 65 (49%) sequential patients having an ICD10 psychiatric diagnosis, most commonly depression. The Hospital Anxiety and Depression scale (HADS) had a good negative predictive value for depression. Moreover, having a psychiatric diagnosis with targeted management was not associated with a better asthma outcome. In a further study in the Brompton cohort, 33 of 56 (58%) subjects had a psychiatric component to their asthma and in 10, this was identified as 'major' (defined as 30% of symptomatic episodes related to feeling tense or subjects said this was 'why I get breathless'). In general, most case-control and observational studies have shown an association between psychological morbidity and difficult to control asthma, although this has not been universal. However, it remains unclear if a 'cause' or 'effect' relationship exists between this observed psychological morbidity and difficult asthma and whether treatment of co-existent psychiatric morbidity improves asthma outcome. In addition, while acute stress and depression are often identified by patients as triggers to their asthma, the impact of these psychological factors on asthma control may manifest as poor adherence with prescribed therapy, rather than a direct effect on asthma severity.

Many patients with asthma have co-existent allergic rhinitis or sinus disease. Again, a pragmatic approach is to give a trial of nasal steroid/anti-histamine for symptomatic nasal disease and if there is a failure of therapy then formal ear nose and throat examination should be arranged. In some patients, managing nasal disease—medically and/or surgically—can have a significant benefit on overall symptom control.

Although the incidence of gastro-oesophageal reflux disease is higher in asthmatic patients than the general population, there is no convincing evidence to support improved asthma control with anti-reflux strategies. Continuous oral prednisolone has been shown to increase gastro-oesophageal reflux disease, and this may exacerbate the problem in 'difficult' asthmatics. Again, a pragmatic approach is to give a trial of standard therapy (proton pump inhibition such as omeprazole or lansoprazole) if symptomatic reflux is present, but evidence for an aggressive investigative strategy for 'silent reflux' with pH profiling is lacking.

Systemic diseases such as thyrotoxicosis, carcinoid syndrome and Churg-Strauss syndrome may cause poor asthma control and should be considered as part of a detailed evaluation. Obstructive sleep apnoea may be more common, particularly in subjects with systemic steroids and should be considered and managed.

A number of medications may worsen asthma control, including beta-blockers (including topical eye drops), NSAIDs and aspirin. These drugs are commonly avoided by asthmatic patients and alternative agents should be used. Occupational factors may play a part in poor disease control, although many patients with difficult asthma have stopped work because of symptoms. Exposure to inhaled allergens (house dust mite, fungal allergens, cat, etc.) can be an important driving factor in persistent asthma symptoms, and changes in living conditions or acquisition of a new pet should be identified with a thorough history. Although there is a relative lack of evidence supporting avoidance of house dust mite and other ubiquitous allergens, removal of pets, if sensitized, seems appropriate (although this advice is frequently ignored).

14.3 True 'therapy-resistant' asthma

Therapy resistant asthma or refractory asthma is present when patients have persisting symptoms despite high dose ICSs (2000 µg beclometasone equivalent) plus long acting β_2-agonists with either maintenance systemic steroids or at least two rescue courses of steroids over 12 months and despite trials of other add-on therapies. This term assumes that the patient has been systematically evaluated and issues mentioned earlier have been addressed. In general, t lowing systematic evaluation and a detailed analysis of all the issue. one-third to a half of patients referred with 'difficult asthma' will not have therapy resistant disease.

Complete steroid resistance is uncommon, and patients with therapy resistance are 'relatively' steroid resistant and will generally respond to higher doses of treatment, usually given systemically. In subjects requiring unacceptable doses of systemic steroids, a trial of an immunosuppressive agent is often given, principally as a steroid sparing medication, though the evidence for benefit is small. The most commonly used immunosuppressive agents for refractory asthma are ciclosporin and methotrexate, although they have a significant side effect profile and limited effectiveness.

Anti Ig-E therapy has a role in a proportion of patients with refractory asthma. An Italian study led by Pace et al. reported improved FEV_1, reduced symptom score and asthma exacerbations in addition to reduced antibiotic, steroid and bronchodilator use in patients treated with omalizumab for seven years, with improvements noted following four years of treatment.

More recently, the RISA (Research in Severe Asthma) Trial Study Group evaluated the use of bronchial thermoplasty in patients with severe asthma. Despite an initial increase in asthma morbidity (transient increase in asthma symptoms, some requiring hospitalization), patients with severe asthma treated with bronchial thermoplasty had reduced rescue medication use and an improvement in FEV_1 and Asthma Control Questionnaire score compared to the control group. At present, 5-year follow up of patients with moderate to severe asthma does not suggest any longer term adverse effects from bronchial thermoplasty.

It is important to assess all difficult asthmatic patients for the presence of osteoporosis with DEXA scanning as many patients will have had considerable systemic steroid exposure. Patients should be prescribed calcium and vitamin D supplements or bisphosphonate treatment, in accordance with appropriate management guidelines, particularly for patients requiring frequent 'bursts' of, or maintenance, systemic steroids.

Further research into alternative asthma therapy for these patients is important due to the significant side-effects of long term oral prednisolone. In order to identify the mechanisms which underpin therapy resistant asthma it is important to ensure that patients included in both mechanistic and therapeutic research programmes are well-characterized. This is most likely to be achieved through the use of systematic evaluation protocols at specialist centres.

14.4 **Conclusion**

When faced with a patient with seemingly 'difficult asthma' it is important to adopt a systematic approach to identify factors contributing to persisting symptoms as summarized in Figure 14.1. This approach is essential before a patient is labelled as having refractory asthma and is considered for new and expensive therapies. Appropriate management of these factors will allow many patients with 'difficult asthma' to be maintained on standard doses of inhaled medication or in some cases, complete withdrawal of treatment if they do not have asthma. Patients with true 'therapy-resistant' asthma usually require high dose asthma treatment and careful clinical follow-up.

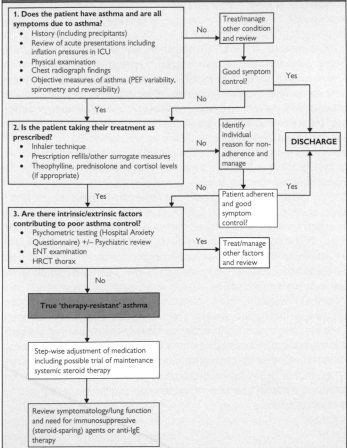

Figure 14.1 Flow chart depicting systemic approach to patient with 'difficult asthma'

Further reading

Barnes PJ, Woolcock AJ (1998) Difficult asthma. *Eur Respir J* **12**: 1209–18

Gamble J, Stevenson M, Heaney LG (2011) A study of a multi-level intervention to improve non-adherence in difficult to control asthma. *Respir Med* Epub ahead of print.

Heaney LG, Conway E, Kelly C, Johnston BT, English C, Stevenson M, Gamble J (2003) Predictors of therapy resistant asthma: outcome of a systematic evaluation protocol. *Thorax* **58**: 561–6.

Moore WC, Meyers DA, Wenzel SE, Teague WG, Li H, Li X et al. (2010) Identification of asthma phenotypes using cluster analysis in the Severe Asthma Research Program. *Am J Respir Crit Care Med* **181**: 315–23.

Pace E, Ferraro M, Bruno A, Chiappara G, Bousquet J, Gjomarkaj M (2011) Clinical benefits of 7 years of treatment with omalizumab in severe uncontrolled asthmatics. *J Asthma* **48**: 387–92.

Robinson DS, Campbell DA, Durham SR, Pfeffer J, Barnes PJ, Chung KF (2003) Systematic assessment of difficult-to-treat asthma. *Eur Respir J* **22**: 478–83.

Ten Brinke A, Ouwerkerk ME, Spinhoven P (2001) Similar psychological characteristics in mild and severe asthma. *J Psychosomatic Res* **50**: 7–10.

Thomson NC, Rubin AS, Niven RM, Corris PA, Siersted HC, Olivenstein R, Pavord ID, McCormack D, Laviolette M, Shargill NS, Cox G (2011) Long-term (5 year) safety of bronchial thermoplasty: Asthma Intervention Research (AIR) trial; AIR Trial Study Group. *BMC Pulm Med* **11**: 11.

Wamboldt MZ, Fritz G, Mansell A, McQuaid EL, Klein RB (1998) Relationship of asthma severity and psychological problems in children. *J Am Acad Child Adolesc Psych* **37**: 943–50.

Index

A

abortions, induced or spontaneous 92
accident and emergency departments, attendance at 71
children 107, 108
reduction through action plans 28
Accuhalers 57, 60, 61
acrylics and acrylates 80
action plans 28–9
allergen avoidance 30–1
altering therapy 29
complementary techniques 31–2
dietary intervention 31
education programmes 28
exacerbations, acute 76, 111
paediatric asthma 111, 114, 120
primary care 127
smoking cessation 32–5
what to do and how long to do it 30
acupuncture 31
acute exacerbations see exacerbations, acute
ADAM33 10
adenoidal hypertrophy/ hyperplasia 102, 104
adenosine monophosphate 20
adherence see compliance
ADRB2 10
adrenocortical suppression 120
aetiology
exacerbations, acute 66–7, 108
occupational asthma 80
paediatric asthma 96–8, 108
Africa, rural/urban differences in prevalence of asthma 2
age factors 2
difficult asthma 132
exacerbations, acute 65–6
mortality 3, 65, 66, 107
paediatric asthma 108, 117–18
see also older patients; paediatric asthma

aggravating factors 14, 135–6
air pollution 11–12
exacerbations, acute 66, 108
paediatric asthma 97, 108
AIR Trial 137
airway hyperresponsiveness to bronchoconstrictor stimuli 38
airway remodelling 8–9
alcalase 81
allergen avoidance
action plans 30–1
difficult asthma 136
paediatric asthma 120–1
allergen exposure 10
difficult asthma 136
exacerbations, acute 66, 108, 119
paediatric asthma 108, 119
allergic alveolitis, extrinsic 134
allergic bronchopulmonary aspergillosis 24–5
allergic rhinitis (hay fever) 22
asthma secondary to 16, 22
in children 96, 98, 99, 102
difficult asthma 136
temporal trends 3, 4
diagnosis 15–16
leukotriene receptor antagonists 46
omalizumab 51
allergy 9, 10, 11
children 96, 97, 98, 102
altering therapy, and action plans 29
alternative medicine 31–2
alveolitis, extrinsic allergic 134
amines 81
aminophylline 74
paediatric asthma 109, 111
pregnancy 92
amylase 80
anaesthesia
in labour 92
paediatric acute exacerbations 111
angiogenesis 5, 6
animals

allergen avoidance 30, 31, 136
difficult asthma 136
occupational asthma 11, 80
paediatric asthma 102, 108, 119
antibiotics 74, 109
anti-cholinergics 51
antidepressants 34
antifungals 24
anti-immunoglobulin E 51, 137
antimalarials 34
antioxidants 11, 97
antipsychotics 34
anxiety 119
apples 11
arachidonic acid 23
arterial blood gases, and acute exacerbations 69
Asia, prevalence of asthma in 2
Aspergillus fumigatus 24
aspirin-sensitive asthma 23
difficult asthma 136
exacerbations, acute 66
leukotriene receptor antagonists 46
assessment
of asthma control 38–9
in pregnancy 89
in primary care 126–7
of paediatric asthma 109, 110
asthma control questionnaire 38, 137
asthma control test 38
asthmagens, occupational 80, 81, 83
asthma therapy assessment questionnaire 38
atomizers 121
atopic eczema see eczema
Australia, prevalence of asthma in 2, 96
Autohalers 57, 60, 63–4

B

bacterial bronchitis 103
bacterial causes, acute exacerbations 66, 74
bakers 11, 80, 83
basement membrane, thickening of the 5, 6
B-carotene 11

141

beclometasone 40
combined inhalers
(Fostair) 44, 45
pregnancy 91
reversibility
testing 17–18
β_2 adrenoceptors 115, 116
β_2 agonists
action plans 30
adverse effects 42–3
bronchial challenge
testing 21
exacerbations,
acute 71–3, 76
paediatric asthma 109
and inhaled corticoster-
oids 42, 43–4
intravenous 73
long-acting
(LABA) 42–3
adverse effects 42–3
and inhaled corticos-
teroids 42, 43–4
occupational asthma 83
paediatric asthma
116–17, 118
pregnancy 90, 92
Symbicort 'SMART'
regime 45
occupational asthma 84
paediatric asthma 115,
116–17, 118, 119
exacerbations,
acute 109
pregnancy 90, 92
reactive airways dysfunc-
tion syndrome 84
reversibility
testing 17–18
short-acting 39–40
action plans 30
bronchial challenge
testing 21
occupational
asthma 83
paediatric asthma 115,
119
reversibility
testing 17–18
Symbicort 'SMART'
regime 45
β blockers 66, 136
betamethasone 91
biological washing
powders 80
biomarkers see inflammatory
biomarkers
birth order 96, 97
breastfeeding 91, 93
paediatric asthma 96, 98
breath activated metered
dose inhalers 62–4
advantages and
disadvantages 57
minimum inspiratory
flow rates 62

paediatric asthma 120
breathlessness,
dysfunctional 133
British Thoracic Society
(BTS) 38
primary care 123,
124, 126
underwater diving
guidelines 93
brittle asthma 23
bronchial challenge
testing 20–1
contraindicated in
pregnancy 88
occupational
asthma 82–3
paediatric asthma 104
reactive airways
dysfunction
syndrome 84
bronchial
hyperresponsiveness/
hyperreactivity 8
paediatric asthma 98
bronchial thermoplasty 53
therapy-resistant
asthma 137
bronchiectasis 133
bronchitis
bacterial 103
chronic 134
bronchiolitis,
obliterative 134
bronchomalacia 103
BTS see British Thoracic
Society
budesonide 40
combined inhalers
(Symbicort®) 43,
44, 45
paediatric asthma 115,
116, 117
pregnancy 91
building industry
workers 80
bupropion 32, 34, 35
Buteyko technique 31
butter 11

C

candidiasis,
oropharyngeal 59
carbamazepine 50, 75
carcinoid syndrome 136
cardiomyopathy 134
cats
allergen avoidance 30, 31
difficult asthma 136
paediatric asthma 102,
108
CD4+ T-helper (Th)
lymphocytes 5, 6–7
CD4+CD25+FoxP3+
T-cells 7
CD8 T-cells 7

cervical ripening 92
chemical process
workers 80
chemokines 8
chest drains 70
chest radiography
allergic
bronchopulmonary
aspergillosis 24, 25
diagnosis of asthma 22
exacerbations, acute 70,
89
pregnancy 89
childbirth 89, 92
children see paediatric
asthma
Children's Asthma Control
Test 114
China, prevalence of asthma
in 2
chlorine gas 84
chrome compounds 80
chronic obstructive
pulmonary
disease (COPD)
bronchial challenge
testing 20–1
differential diagnosis 15,
16, 133
tiotropium 51
viral induced
wheeze 105
Churg–Strauss
syndrome 24
difficult asthma 136
leukotriene receptor
antagonists 46–8
chymase 8
ciclesonide 40, 41, 42
cigarette smoking 10
bronchial challenge
testing 20–1
cessation 32
adolescents 121
behavioural
support 32
bupropion 34, 35
nicotine replacement
therapy 33–4
in pregnancy 33, 90
varenicline 34–5
chronic obstructive
pulmonary disease 15
maternal 32, 98
paediatric asthma 32,
96, 97, 119, 121
maternal
smoking 32, 98
in pregnancy 10, 88
cessation 33, 90
reviewing smoking status
in primary care 128
ciliary dyskinesia 103
ciprofloxacin 49, 75
clarithromycin 49,
51, 75

classical occupational
asthma 79, 80
causes 80
clinical features 81
diagnosis 82–3
legal issues 85
management 83
pathogenesis 81
prognosis 84
cleaners 81
cleft palate 91
clinical features 14–16
exacerbations,
acute 67–9
occupational asthma 81
in pregnancy 89
cold, common
(rhinovirus) 97, 105, 108
'cold freon' effect 59
colophony 11, 80
combination inhalers 43–4
dosing regime 44
paediatric asthma 118
common cold
(rhinovirus) 97, 105, 108
complementary
medicine 31–2
compliance
difficult asthma 134, 135
exacerbations,
acute 71, 111
paediatric asthma 111,
115, 116, 117, 118–19
in pregnancy 88
psychological
morbidity 135
Control of Substances
Hazardous to
Health (COSHH)
regulations 83
coolants 80
COPD see chronic
obstructive pulmonary
disease
corticosteroids
action plans 30
adverse effects 42, 50,
52, 120
allergic bronchopulmo-
nary aspergillosis 24
Churg–Strauss
syndrome 24
cough variant asthma 23
difficult asthma 132, 134
exacerbations,
acute 73, 76
paediatric
asthma 109, 111
inhaled 40–2
action plans 30
adverse effects 42, 120
Churg–Strauss
syndrome 24
cough variant
asthma 23
difficult asthma 134

eosinophilic
bronchitis 23
exacerbations,
acute 109
and long-acting β_2
agonists 42, 43, 45
metered dose
inhalers 59
occupational
asthma 83
paediatric asthma 104,
109, 115–17, 118–19,
120
pregnancy 90, 91, 92
reversibility
testing 17–18
smoking 32
intravenous 73
and long-acting β_2
agonists 42, 43, 45
metered dose
inhalers 59
occupational asthma 83
oral 50
action plans 30
adverse effects 50, 52
Churg–Strauss
syndrome 24
difficult asthma 132,
134
exacerbations,
acute 73, 76, 109,
111
paediatric asthma 109,
111, 117, 118
peak expiratory flow
rate variability 18–19
pregnancy 90, 91–2
reversibility
testing 17–18
paediatric asthma 104,
115–17, 118–19
adverse effects 120
exacerbations,
acute 109, 111
and viral induced
wheeze, differential
diagnosis 105
peak expiratory flow
rate variability 18–19
pregnancy 90, 91–2
reactive airways
dysfunction
syndrome 84
reversibility
testing 17–18
smoking 32
therapy-resistant
asthma 132, 137
cortisol, plasma levels
of 134
COSHH regulations 83
costs of asthma 4–5, 65, 84
cough
paediatric asthma 102,
103

reactive airways dysfunc-
tion syndrome 84
cough variant asthma 23
Creola bodies 5
croup 102
cutting oils 80
cyclo-oxygenase-1 23
ciclosporin 53, 119, 137
cysteinyl leukotrienes 23,
46
cystic fibrosis 103, 134
cytokines 8, 67

D

day care, and paediatric
asthma 96
death see mortality
definition of asthma 1–2
dehumidifiers 121
dehydration 76
depression 35, 135
desisobutyryl-
ciclesonide 40, 41
dexamethasone 91
diagnosis 13–14
allergic
bronchopulmonary
aspergillosis 24–5
allergic rhinitis 22
aspirin-sensitive
asthma 23
brittle asthma 23
bronchial challenge
testing 20–1
chest radiograph 22
Churg–Strauss
syndrome 24
cough variant asthma 23
differential 14–16
in children 104–5
difficult
asthma 133–14
in pregnancy 88, 89
eosinophilic
bronchitis 23
exercise testing 19
full blood count 22
IgE level 22
inflammatory
biomarkers 21–2
occupational
asthma 82–3
paediatric asthma 101
exacerbations,
acute 108
history 101–4
physiological
testing 104
viral induced
wheeze 104–5
in pregnancy 88–9
in primary care 124–5
RAST 22
reactive airways dysfunc-
tion syndrome 84

diagnosis (cont.)
reversibility
testing 17–18
signs 16
skin prick tests 22
spirometry 16–17
variability in peak
expiratory flow 18–19
dialdehydes 81
dicarboxylic acid
anhydrides 81
diet
action plans 31
maternal, during
pregnancy 96
paediatric asthma 96,
97, 98
as risk factor 11
differential diagnosis 14–16
in children 104–5
difficult asthma 133–14
in pregnancy 88, 89
difficult asthma 131–6, 138
therapy-resistant
asthma 136–7
discharge planning 76, 111
dispensing costs 5
diurnal variations in PEF 19
brittle asthma 23
exacerbations, acute 76
in pregnancy 89
diving 93
dogs 30, 31, 102, 108
drug treatment see pharmacological management
dry powder inhalers
(DPIs) 60–2
advantages and
disadvantages 57
paediatric asthma 120
dysfunctional
breathlessness 133
dysphonia 59
dyspnoea of pregnancy 88

E

early origins hypothesis 97
Easibreathe inhalers 57,
60, 62–3
economic costs of
asthma 4–5, 65, 84
eczema
diagnosis 15, 16
paediatric asthma 96,
98, 99, 102
temporal trends 3, 4
education programmes 28
difficult asthma 134
exacerbations,
prevention of 77, 111
paediatric asthma 111
pregnancy 90
primary care 127
elderly patients 56, 93
electrolyte imbalance 76

electroplaters 80
emergency treatment 4
see also exacerbations,
acute
engineers 80
environmental pollution
11–12
exacerbations,
acute 66, 108
paediatric asthma 97, 108
enzymes 80, 81
eosinophil cationic protein 7
eosinophilia 6
sputum 21, 22, 23, 38
eosinophilic bronchitis 23
eosinophils 5, 6, 7–8
allergic
bronchopulmonary
aspergillosis 24
Churg–Strauss
syndrome 24
full blood count 22
mast cell activation 8
eotaxin 7
epidemiology 2–5
exacerbations,
acute 65–6, 107–8
paediatric asthma 96,
107–8
epilepsy 34
epithelial disruption 5, 6
airway remodelling 9
paediatric asthma 98
epoxy resin workers 81
erythromycin 49, 75
exacerbations, acute 65
action plans 28
admission to hospital 71
aetiology 66–7, 108
clinical features 67–9
discharge planning 76, 111
epidemiology 65–6,
107–8
flying 93
investigations 69–70
management 71–6,
109–11, 115
paediatric asthma
aetiology 108
assessment 109
discharge planning 111
epidemiology 107–8
management 109–11,
115
prevention 111
pathogenesis 67
in pregnancy 71, 88,
89, 90–2
prevention 77, 111
exercise-induced
asthma 46, 108
exercise testing 19, 20
underwater diving 93
exhaled nitric oxide
see nitric oxide,
exhaled

extrinsic allergic
alveolitis 134

F

family history 15, 102
'farming effect' 10
fatty acids 11
FCER1B 10
feathers 30, 121
fetal origins hypothesis 97
FEV₁ see forced expiratory
volume in 1 second
FEV₁/FVC ratio 16
financial costs of
asthma 4–5, 65, 84
fish oil supplementation 31
5-lipoxygenase pathway 23
'floppy airway' 103
flour 11, 80, 83
flu 121
fluticasone 40
combined inhalers
(Seretide®) 43–4
paediatric asthma 115,
116, 117
pregnancy 91
fluxes 11
flying 93–4
food allergy 96, 102
Food and Drug
Administration 43
forced expiratory volume in
1 second (FEV₁) 16, 17
bronchial challenge
testing 20–1
bronchial
thermoplasty 137
FEV₁/FVC ratio 16
occupational asthma 82–3
paediatric asthma 99
pregnancy 89
reversibility testing 17–18
underwater diving 93
forced vital capacity
(FVC) 16, 17
foreign body, aspiration of
a 103, 108
formoterol 42
combined inhalers
(Fostair, Symbicort®)
44, 45, 92
pregnancy 92
Fostair 45
free radicals 7
fruit juice 11
full blood count 22
fungal allergens 136
FVC (forced vital
capacity) 16, 17

G

γδ cells 7
gastro-oesophageal reflux
disease 23, 136

gender factors 3
  difficult asthma 132
  paediatric asthma 96, 98
general anaesthesia during
  labour 92
general practitioners (GPs)
  costs of consultations 5
  exacerbations, acute 76,
   107
  numbers of
   consultations 4
  paediatric asthma 107
  reduction in hospital
   admissions 28
  see also primary care
genetic factors 9–10, 15,
  96, 115
geographical differences 2
Germany, reunification
  of 2, 97
glutaraldehyde asthma 83
goals of asthma
  management 27
goblet cell hyperplasia 5, 6
gold 53
GPRA 10
GPs see general
  practitioners
grain dust 11, 80
'grandmother' effect 10
grass 102, 108, 121
growth, and paediatric
  asthma 96, 120

H

haptens 81
hay fever see allergic rhinitis
healthcare professionals
  education
   opportunities 28
  occupational asthma 11,
   81, 83
  training 128
heparin 76
herbal preparations 31
Hippocrates 95
histamine
  bronchial challenge
   testing 20–1, 82–3
  mast cell activation 8
histopathology 5, 6
historical background to
  asthma 95
history taking
  difficult asthma 136
  occupational asthma 81
  paediatric
   asthma 101–2, 104
  primary care 125
homeopathy 31
hospital admissions and visits
  costs 5, 65
  discharge planning 76,
   111
  epidemiology 65–6

management 71–6
paediatric asthma 107,
  111
pregnancy 71, 89
rates 4, 65
reduction
  through action
   plans 28
  through GP contacts 28
Hospital Anxiety and
  Depression Scale
  (HADS) 135
house dust mite 10, 30
  difficult asthma 136
  paediatric asthma 98, 108
humidifiers 121
hydrocortisone 73, 92, 125
hygiene hypothesis 10–11,
  97
hypereosinophilia 134
hypermagnesaemia 74
hypertonic saline 20, 21
hyperventilation
  syndrome 133
hypotension 90–1
hypoxia
  exacerbations, acute 71,
   90–1
  flying 93–4
  pregnancy 90–1

I

IgA deficiency 134
IgE see immunoglobulin E
IL-10 6, 7
IL-13 6
IL-4 6, 7
IL-5 6, 7
IL-6 6
IL-9 6
immediate hypersensitivity
  reaction 8, 9
immunity in pregnancy 88
immunoglobulin A (IgA)
  deficiency 134
immunoglobulin E (IgE) 6,
  7, 8
  allergen exposure 10
  allergic
   bronchopulmomary
   aspergillosis 24, 25
  anti-IgE 51, 137
  Churg–Strauss
   syndrome 24
  diagnosis of asthma 22
  occupational asthma 81
immunosuppressants 24,
  51, 137
immunotherapy 121
impact of asthma 3–5
inactivity 11, 97
incidence of asthma 4
India, prevalence of
  asthma in 2
induced abortion 92

inflammation of the
  airways 5
  obesity 11
inflammatory
  biomarkers 21–2, 38–9
  paediatric asthma 104
influenza 121
inhaled corticosteroids see
  under corticosteroids
inhalers 55–8
  advantages and
   disadvantages of
   different types 57
  flying 93
  ideal attributes 58
  paediatric
   asthma 119–20
  prescription filling
   as compliance
   measurement 134
  technique
   Accuhalers 61
   assessment 28, 56, 111
   Autohalers 63
   correction 56
   Easibreathe
    inhalers 62–3
   metered dose
    inhalers 58–9
   metered dose inhalers
    plus spacers 59–60
   paediatric asthma 111,
    119–20
   Turbohalers 62
  types 58–64
intensive care units 75–6, 90
intercellular adhesion
  molecule 1 (ICAM-1) 7
interleukins 6, 7
International Study of
  Asthma and Allergy in
  Children 96
invasive ventilation 70, 75–6
ipratropium
  exacerbations, acute 73,
   109, 111
  paediatric asthma 109,
   111, 115
isocyanates 11, 80, 81, 84
isolation, social 71
itraconazole 24

L

laboratory animal
  proteins 80
labour 89, 92
lactation 91, 93
  paediatric asthma 96, 98
lansoprazole 136
laryngomalacia 103
late phase reaction 8, 9, 81
latent period, occupational
  asthma 81
latex 11, 80, 83

legal issues, occupational asthma 85
leukotriene receptor antagonists (LTRAs) 46–8
adverse effects 46–8
aspirin-sensitive asthma 23
Churg–Strauss syndrome 24
exacerbations, acute 74–5
paediatric asthma 111, 116–17, 118
pregnancy 90, 92
leukotrienes 8, 74
5-lipoxygenase pathway 23
lithium 50, 75
long-acting β_2 agonists see under β_2 agonists
low molecular weight heparin 76
low self-esteem 119
lumbar anaesthesia during labour 92
lymphocytes 5, 6–7, 8

M

macrolides 51
magnesium 31, 73–4
paediatric asthma 109, 111
pregnancy 92
major basic protein 7
management of asthma see non-pharmacological management; pharmacological management
management plans see action plans
mannitol 20
margarine 11
mast cells 6, 7, 8
mastocytosis 6
medication see pharmacological management
metered dose inhalers (MDIs) 58–9
advantages and disadvantages 57
breath activated metered dose inhalers 62–4
advantages and disadvantages 57
minimum inspiratory flow rates 62
paediatric asthma 120
introduction 55
with spacers 59–60
advantages and disadvantages 57
paediatric asthma 109, 119–20

sub-optimal delivery 56
methacholine, bronchial challenge
testing 20, 21
contraindicated in pregnancy 88
occupational asthma 82–3
reactive airways dysfunction syndrome 84
methotrexate 53, 137
methylxanthines 48–9, 50, 74, 92
migratory populations 2
mineral supplementation 31
montelukast 46
chemical structure 47
paediatric asthma 116–17
prescribing and pharmacokinetic data 48
morbidity 4
psychosocial/ psychiatric 135
mortality
age factors 3, 65, 66, 107
long-acting β_2 agonists 43
oral corticosteroids, immediate withdrawal after prolonged administration 50
paediatric asthma 107
psychosocial morbidity 135
risk factors 66–7
seasonal factors 65
in the UK 3, 65, 66
mucus gland hypertrophy 5, 6
mucus plugs 5, 6
mucus production, increased 5, 6

N

NAEPP 132
National Asthma Education and Prevention Program 132
National Institute for Health and Clinical Excellence 51
natural killer cells 7
nebulizers 64
advantages and disadvantages 57
exacerbations, acute 71–3, 76, 109–11, 115
flying 93
paediatric asthma 109–11, 115, 120
neonates 10

New Zealand, prevalence of asthma in 2, 96
NICE 51
nicotine replacement therapy (NRT) 32, 33–4
nitric oxide, exhaled 21, 22, 38, 39
paediatric asthma 104
nitrogen oxides 11, 12, 108
non-invasive ventilation (NIV) 75
non-pharmacological management 27
action plans 28–9
allergen avoidance 30–1
altering therapy 29
complementary techniques 31–2
dietary intervention 31
smoking cessation 32–5
what to do and for how long 30
education programmes 28
occupational asthma 83
paediatric asthma 120–1
pregnancy 90
non-steroidal anti-inflammatory drugs 66, 136
NSAIDs 66, 136
nuts 102

O

OASYS 82–3
obesity and overweight 11
dietary intervention 31
difficult asthma 132
paediatric asthma 96, 97, 121
in pregnancy 88
obliterative bronchiolitis 134
obstructive sleep apnoea 134, 136
occupational asthma 11, 79
causes 80
classical 80–4
clinical features 81
diagnosis 18, 82–3
difficult asthma 136
exacerbations, acute 66
legal issues 85
management 83
pathogenesis 81
prognosis 84
reactive airways dysfunction syndrome 84
variability in PEF 18
work-aggravated asthma 84

olamizumab 119
older patients 56, 93
omalizumab 51, 137
omega 3 fatty acids 33
omeprazole 136
oral corticosteroids *see
under* corticosteroids
oropharyngeal
candidiasis 59
osteoporosis,
corticosteroid-
induced 50, 137
overweight *see* obesity and
overweight
oxides of nitrogen 11,
12, 108
oxygen
exacerbations, acute 71,
76, 109
flying 93–4
paediatric asthma 109
pregnancy 90
primary care 125
ozone 108

P

$PaCO_2$ 69
paediatric asthma 95
aetiology 96–8
beyond childhood 99
chronic
management 113–17
age factors 118
goals 114
ineffective 118–19
inhalers 119–20
non-therapeutic 120–1
side effects 120
stepping down and
stopping
treatment 119
diagnosis 101
exacerbations,
acute 108
history 101–4
physiological
testing 104
viral induced
wheeze 104–5
epidemiology 2–3, 96
exacerbations, acute
aetiology 108
assessment 109, 110
diagnosis 108
discharge planning 111
epidemiology 107–8
management 109–11
prevention 111
historical backdrop 95
hospital visits 65
impact 4
natural history 98–9
outdoor air
pollution 12
phenotypes 98–9

physiological and
pathological
changes 98
prevalence 3
paint spraying 11, 80, 81
p anti-neutrophil
cytoplasmic antibody
(pANCA) 24
PaO_2 69
paracetamol 97
particulates 11, 108
pastry makers 11
pathogenesis 98
exacerbations, acute 67
occupational asthma 81
pathology 5–6, 98
pathophysiology 3, 6–9, 98
PC_{20} (provocation
concentration),
bronchial challenge
testing 20, 21
pCO_2 69
PD_{20} (provocation dose),
bronchial challenge
testing 20, 21
peak expiratory flow (PEF)
action plans 29
brittle asthma 23
diurnal variations in 19
brittle asthma 24
exacerbations,
acute 76
in pregnancy 89
exacerbations,
acute 68, 76
discharge planning 76
hospital admissions 71
exercise testing 19
monitoring asthma
control 28
occupational
asthma 82, 83
paediatric
asthma 104, 114
pregnancy 88–9
reversibility
testing 17–18
underwater diving 93
variability in 18–19
peak flow meters 18, 19
PEF *see* peak expiratory
flow
personal protective
equipment, occupational
asthma 83
pertussis 103
pets
allergen avoidance 30, 31
difficult asthma 136
paediatric asthma 102,
108
pH, arterial blood gas 69
pharmacological
management 37–8
anti-cholinergics 51
anti-IgE 51

assessment of asthma
control 38–9
and breastfeeding 93
bronchial
thermoplasty 53
costs 5
immunosuppressants
51–3
inhaled
corticosteroids 40–2
leukotriene receptor
antagonists 46–8
long-acting β_2
agonists 42–5
macrolides 51
methylxanthines 48–50,
92
occupational asthma 83
oral corticosteroids 50
adverse effects 52
paediatric
asthma 114–20
exacerbations,
acute 109–11
in pregnancy 90–2
compliance 88
primary care 125
reactive airways
dysfunction
syndrome 84
short-acting β_2
agonists 39–40
see also specific drugs
phenotypes 97, 98–9, 132
phenytoin 49, 75
plumbers 80
pneumothorax 70
pO_2 69
pollution 11–12
exacerbations, acute 66,
108
paediatric asthma 97, 108
polyunsaturated fatty
acids 11
post-nasal drip
syndrome 23
postpartum
haemorrhage 92
practice nurses 76
pranlukast 46
prednisolone 50
adverse effects 50,
52, 137
difficult asthma 136
exacerbations,
acute 73, 76
paediatric
asthma 109, 111
flying 93
gastro-oesophageal
reflux disease 136
labour 92
plasma levels,
measurement 134
pregnancy 91, 92
primary care 125

prednisolone (*cont.*)
  reversibility
    testing 17–18, 19
  therapy-resistant
    asthma 137
prednisone 50
pregnancy 87–8
  clinical features of
    asthma 89
  diagnosis of
    asthma 88–9
  diet during 11, 96, 97
  exacerbations, acute 88,
    89, 90–2
    hospital admission 71,
      89
  'farming effect' 10
  fetal origins hypothesis,
    paediatric asthma 97
  hygiene hypothesis 10–11
  and leukotriene receptor
    antagonists 46
  management of
    asthma 90–1, 91–2
    β_2 agonists 91–2
    inhaled
      corticosteroids 91
    in labour 92
    leukotriene receptor
      antagonists 92
    oral
      corticosteroids 91–2
  smoking during 10, 88
    cessation 33, 90
pressurized metered dose
  inhalers (pMDIs) 58–9
  advantages and
    disadvantages 57
  breath activated
    metered dose
    inhalers 62–4
    advantages and
      disadvantages 57
    minimum inspiratory
      flow rates 62
    paediatric asthma 120
  introduction 55
  with spacers 59–60
    advantages and
      disadvantages 57
    paediatric asthma 109,
      119–20
  sub-optimal delivery 56
prevalence of asthma 2, 3
  aspirin-sensitive 23
  paediatric asthma 96,
    107
  in the UK 3, 96, 107
primary care 123
  contract 123–4
  diagnosis 124–5
  management 125
  practice nurses 76
  Quality Outcomes
    Framework 123–4,
    125, 126, 127
  limitations 128–9

record keeping 126
referrals 126
review 126–8
staff development 128
websites 129
see also general
  practitioners
probability of
  asthma 13–14, 17, 18
prostaglandins 8, 92
protective equipment,
  occupational asthma 83
provocation dose/
  concentration (PD$_{20}$/
  PC$_{20}$), bronchial
  challenge testing 20, 21
provoking stimuli 14, 135–6
psychiatric morbidity 135
pulmonary embolism 88
pulmonary
  hypertension 134
pulsus paradoxus 69, 109

Q

Quality Outcomes
  Framework
  (QOF) 123–4, 125,
  126, 127
  limitations 128–9
questionnaires to assess
  asthma control 38
quinolones 34

R

radioallergosorbent test
  (RAST) 22, 24
rattle 102, 103
rat urine 80
reactive airways dysfunction
  syndrome (RADS)
  79, 84
record keeping in primary
  care 126
referrals 126
refractory
  (therapy-resistant)
  asthma 132, 136–7, 138
regional anaesthesia during
  labour 92
relaxation techniques 32, 90
remodelling of airways 8–9
Reporting of Injuries,
  Diseases and Dangerous
  Occurrences
  Regulations
  (RIDDOR) 83
Research in Severe Asthma
  (RISA) 137
respiratory failure 69
respiratory muscle
  incoordination 134
respiratory tract
  infections 96, 97,
  104–5, 108

reticular basement
  membrane, thickening of
  the 5, 6
reversibility testing 17–18, 19
review appointments,
  primary care 126–8
rhinitis 127, 128
  allergic see allergic
    rhinitis (hay fever)
rhinovirus (common
  cold) 97, 105, 108
RIDDOR 83
rifampicin 49, 75
RISA (Research in Severe
  Asthma) 137
risk factors for
  asthma 9–12
  exacerbations,
    acute 66–7
Royal College of
  Physicians 126
rural/urban differences in
  prevalence of asthma 2
'ruttle' (rattle) 102, 103

S

salbutamol 39
  exacerbations, acute
    71–3, 76, 109, 111
  paediatric asthma 109,
    111, 115
  reversibility
    testing 17–18
saline, hypertonic 20, 21
salmeterol 42
  adverse effects 42–3
  combined inhalers
    (Seretide®) 44, 45, 92
  pregnancy 92
salt, dietary 31
Scottish Intercollegiate
  Guidelines Network
  (SIGN) 123, 124, 126
Scottish Medicines
  Consortium 51
seasonal factors 65, 108
sedentary lifestyle 11, 97
seizures 34
selenium 11
self-esteem, low 119
Seretide® 44, 45
Severe Asthma Research
  Program 132
short-acting β_2 agonists
  see under β_2 agonists
SIGN 123, 124, 126
signs of asthma 16
sinus disease 136
skin prick tests 22
  allergic bronchopulmo-
    nary aspergillosis 24
  paediatric asthma 99, 104
sleep apnoea 134, 136
smoking see cigarette
  smoking

smooth muscle
  hypertrophy/
  proliferation 5, 6
social isolation 71
sodium, dietary 31
solder 80, 81
spacer devices 42, 59–60
  advantages and
    disadvantages 57
  paediatric asthma 109,
    119–20
spirometry 13, 14, 16–17
  paediatric asthma 98,
    104
  pregnancy 88
  reactive airways
    dysfunction
    syndrome 84
  underwater diving 93
SpO$_2$ 69
spontaneous abortion 92
sputum eosinophilia 21,
  22, 23, 38
staff training 128
stepwise management of
  asthma
  in adults 38, 39
  in children 114–18, 119
steroids see corticosteroids
stertor 102, 104
stress 32, 135
stress avoidance
  strategies 32
stridor 102
subtypes of asthma 22–5
suicidal ideation 35
sulphur dioxide 11, 108
Symbicort® 44, 45
  'SMART' regime 45

T

tartrazine 23
temporal trends 3
terbutaline 39, 71, 115
Th1 lymphocytes 6–7
Th2 lymphocytes 5,
  6–7, 8
Th9 lymphocytes 7
Th17 lymphocytes 7
Th22 lymphocytes 7
theophyllines 48–50

adverse effects 49–50
bupropion 34
chemical structure 49
exacerbations,
  acute 74
paediatric asthma 117,
  118
plasma concentration
  factors affecting
    49–50, 75
  measurement 134
pregnancy 90, 92
therapy-resistant
  (refractory) asthma 132,
  136–7, 138
thromboprophylaxis 76
thyrotoxicosis 136
timber workers 11, 80
tiotropium 51
tobacco smoking see
  cigarette smoking
tracheomalacia 103
traffic pollution 12
training, staff 128
treatment of asthma see
  non-pharmacological
  management; pharmaco-
  logical management
tryptase 8
Turbohalers 57, 60, 61–2
twin studies 9, 15, 96

U

underwater diving 93
United Kingdom
  air pollution 11
  COSHH regulations 83
  impact of asthma 3–4, 5
  occupational
    asthma 11, 83
  paediatric asthma
    96, 97
  prevalence of
    asthma 2, 96
  RIDDOR 83
United States Food and
  Drug Administration 43
United States of America
  impact of asthma 5
  prevalence of paediatric
    asthma 96

upper respiratory tract
  infections 96, 97, 104–5,
  108
urban/rural differences in
  prevalence of asthma 2

V

varenicline 32, 34–5
ventilation
  invasive 70, 75–6
  non-invasive
    ventilation 75
verapamil 49, 75
viral causes
  exacerbations, acute 66,
    108
  paediatric asthma 96,
    97, 108
viral induced wheeze 104–5
vitamin C 11
vitamin D 11
vitamin E 11, 97
vitamin supplementation 31
vocal cord dysfunction 103,
  133

W

washing powders 80
weight gain 34
weight loss 31, 121
welders 11, 80
Westernized lifestyle 2
  hygiene hypothesis 10
  obesity 11
  paediatric asthma 96–7
wheeze 102
  viral induced 104–5
wood dust 11, 80
work-aggravated
  asthma 79, 84
World Health
  Organization 132
World Trade Centre 84

Z

zafirlukast 46, 47, 48
zileuton 46
zinc 11